Withdrawn

The Immune Mystery

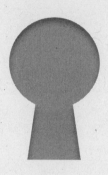

DR. ANITA KÅSS
AND JØRGEN JELSTAD

Translated by
ALISON MCCULLOUGH

THE
IMMUNE
MYSTERY

A Doctor's Impassioned
Quest to Solve the Puzzle
of Autoimmune Disease

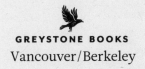

GREYSTONE BOOKS
Vancouver/Berkeley

Greystone Books Ltd.
greystonebooks.com

Cataloguing data available from Library and Archives Canada
ISBN 978-1-77164-550-8 (cloth)
ISBN 978-1-77164-551-5 (epub)

Copy editing by Paula Ayer
Proofreading by Alison Strobel
Indexing by Stephen Ullstrom
Jacket and text design by Fiona Siu

Printed and bound in Canada on ancient-forest-friendly paper by Friesens

This work reflects the ideas and opinions of the author. It aims to provide
useful information on the topics covered in these pages. Neither the author nor the
publisher is offering medical, health, or other professional services in this book. The
author and the publisher are not responsible for any liability, damage, loss, or risk,
whether personal or otherwise, suffered as a result of the direct or indirect use or
application of any element of the contents of this work.

Greystone Books gratefully acknowledges the
Musqueam, Squamish, and Tsleil-Waututh peoples on
whose land our office is located.

Greystone Books thanks the Canada Council for the Arts,
the British Columbia Arts Council, the Province of British Columbia
through the Book Publishing Tax Credit, and the Government of
Canada for supporting our publishing activities.

Canadä

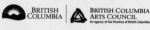

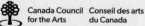

This translation has been published with the financial support of NORLA.

To Dea, Maia, and Ingrid Marie

CONTENTS

PROLOGUE

I STARED AT THE line on the floor. "Just stand here, then walk
out when your name is called," said the man who had posi-
tioned me there. He smiled reassuringly as he listened to the
message being relayed over his huge headphones. On either side
of the TV studio, rows of seats sloped up toward the ceiling. The
laughter from the audience faded among the stage lights, and
applause took over. It would soon be my turn.

This was not my home turf—I preferred to be sitting in my
office full of books and research articles, or to be examining samples under the fancy microscope we had at the hospital. But I was
now about to appear on Scandinavia's biggest talk show. A couple of million viewers were waiting for me out there. What was I
doing here?

The past week had been a hectic one, with journalists calling
me incessantly and my husband finally having to act as my secretary, fielding their inquiries. I didn't have the stamina to respond
to all of them—sharing my life and work in this way was completely alien to me. This was everything I had worked so hard for,
over so many years. Now the same questions would be put to me
again. About the medicine, about the money. About Mum.

The applause abated. On the round stage a few yards away the
talk show host smiled as he looked straight into the camera, took

a breath, and said: "At a small hospital in Norway, a researcher has been working to develop a treatment for rheumatoid arthritis—and possibly psoriasis, multiple sclerosis, and other diseases. Last week, it was announced that the rights for this treatment have been sold for 800 million kroner. Please welcome researcher Anita Kåss!"

I had never been so nervous in my entire life.

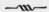

AS I TOOK those first few steps onto the stage, terrified that I might trip and fall, a hormonal storm was raging within me. In situations involving extreme stress, we all experience the more uncomfortable aspects of having a body. We might sweat or shake; feel slightly nauseous or be struck by tingling sensations. Things happen that are beyond our control, and that affect how we feel, what we're able to do—even our very sense of who we are. This discomfort is due to hormones, the body's messengers, working at a frantic pace. They affect cells throughout the entire body, among them billions of faithful soldiers—the army that keeps us alive.

Every day our soldiers go to war. They march and fight, win battles and die—fearless and loyal until their dying breath. To study them under a microscope is to peer into a universe of super-heroes, where each and every one has its own special powers and cool costume. This is the immune system—the world's most sophisticated killing machine.

The body has many systems. The digestive system, consisting of the mouth, esophagus, stomach, and intestines, is easy to understand. Likewise the cardiovascular system, with the heart at its center and its network of blood vessels; or the nervous system, with the brain and its branching nerve fibers. You can point to each of these systems and say: there it is. But where in the body is the army, the immune system, stationed?

The answer is everywhere. In order to defend us against attacks from foreign intruders, this inner army has access to every nook and cranny of the kingdom that is the body. Within this kingdom is everything we need in order to live: energy production, waste disposal, infrastructure and transport, lines of communication, and birthing rooms for cells. To get a person through the events of everyday life demands indefatigable efforts from billions of inhabitants on the inside.

The body is a peaceful land surrounded by dangers; all foreign substances are potential enemies. This is why the body has a military academy that puts its soldiers through the toughest of training camps, and only the very best pass the final test. They patrol our borders and monitor alien intruders, checking them against a comprehensive register in order to find out who they are and whether or not it's safe to let them in.

These soldiers are white blood cells—the cells of the immune system. And although they patrol the entire body, there are certain areas and organs that house large parts of this army. The training camps are located in the bone marrow and in a small organ located just above the heart, known as the thymus. Hundreds of outposts—the lymph nodes—are spread around the body, connected by the lymphatic vessels. If the blood vessels are the roads of this country, then the lymphatic vessels are its sidewalks.

Even with vigilant defenses, intruders often manage to sneak past border patrols and outposts. Suddenly the bus station might be set on fire, or a bomb might be detonated by the waterworks. Hostile terrorists might be spawned within the residential areas of a city.

When this happens, local soldiers quickly launch counterattacks to stop these intruders. Blaring alarms are sounded, and special forces storm the scene to strike the final blow. When the conflict is over, the inhabitants clear and repair the battlefield. And then life carries on more or less as before. But not always.

—⁓—

THIS BOOK DESCRIBES how our spectacular immune system works, and looks at what can happen when things go wrong—how the body's defenses are in fact able to make our existence a chronic nightmare. And how in the most extreme cases, these defenses can destroy us, annihilating the very body that keeps them alive.

When the body attacks itself, we call the condition an autoimmune disease. "Auto" means "self." The immune system attacks "the self." Examples of autoimmune diseases include rheumatoid arthritis, psoriasis, multiple sclerosis, type 1 diabetes, Sjögren's syndrome, celiac disease, inflammatory bowel disease, and ankylosing spondylitis. The list is long—over a hundred diseases are thought to be caused by the body's own soldiers making disastrous mistakes.

Statistically, if you invite ten of your friends to dinner, one of them will suffer from an autoimmune disease. If you attend a wedding with a hundred guests, one of them will have rheumatoid arthritis. And if you're among those who have a thousand friends on Facebook, it's likely that a couple of these will have multiple sclerosis. Autoimmune diseases affect so many people that if you suffer from one yourself, you'll hardly be alone among family and friends. And if you yourself are not affected, you're guaranteed to know someone who is. Many tens of millions of people across the world live year upon year with the consequences of a mistake within their immune system. Autoimmune diseases are one of the most significant causes of death among people under the age of seventy, and particularly among women.

For health care authorities, autoimmune diseases are responsible for some of the largest expenditures in their budgets. For patients, the cost is in some cases a life ruined.

Why the body attacks itself is one of medicine's greatest mysteries. It is also the mystery of my mother—a puzzle I have wanted to solve since childhood. The desire to solve this mystery has led me on a long journey, toward something I hope will help to improve the lives of all those who suffer as my mum did.

BEGINNINGS

"I love the past.
There are parts of the past I hate, of course."
PAUL MCCARTNEY, BORN IN 1942
AT WALTON HOSPITAL, LIVERPOOL

M UM LOOKED OUT at the October rain running down the windowpanes as she passed a hand over her belly. Would tonight be the night? She looked over at Dad and smiled. A new life awaited these two expectant doctors in Liverpool. They would soon be a family.

It wasn't long before they entered the redbrick building that housed Walton Hospital. A birth was far from Dad's everyday life as a psychiatrist, and the careful smile his patients had come to know so well now had a slightly nervous look to it. Unease and worry, pain, smiles, and tears—some hours in life contain everything. But in Mum's body, an unexpected storm was brewing.

I was born on a Monday in 1979. Little did my parents know that this would be the start of years of suffering.

They had married only a year before, back home in India. Dad's family had noticed a newspaper advertisement, and along with one of his brothers, Dad traveled hundreds of miles to the industrial city of Kanpur to find out more about the woman in the ad.

A woman who had qualified as a doctor, and who was strikingly beautiful in her colorful sari. Mum. After just a single meeting they married in my father's home town of Chandigarh.

That same year, they packed their belongings into suitcases and moved to Liverpool, England—a common journey for highly educated Indians seeking a better future. There, they found a small house in the suburb of Rainhill, right next to the Whiston Hospital, where Dad started work. Mum got a job as a pathologist at Royal Liverpool University Hospital, where she spent her days studying tissue samples to look for cancer and taking the occasional trip down to the autopsy room. It wasn't long before she became pregnant.

When two cells merge and start to develop into a baby, there is one system the mother's body must hold in check—the immune system. The patrolling cells of this system quickly notice if anything foreign suddenly appears in their hunting grounds, and a growing fetus might be regarded as an intruder, a potential hazard.

Over millions of years, the body's defenses have developed to attack everything that may pose a threat. But our survival as a species is equally dependent on mothers being able to carry children who are genetically different from themselves. This is the immunological paradox of pregnancy. The immune system is technically incompatible with having children, but something tells it that the fetus must be left alone; without these finely tuned control mechanisms, none of us would have been born. For over fifty years, researchers have tried to find out exactly what happens during these nine months, but we still don't have all the answers as to how the female body controls the cells of its immune system during pregnancy.

Might this paradox help us to understand how autoimmune diseases arise? For Mum, this was exactly where it started—with pregnancy and birth, when something tipped her immune system

7

out of balance. What is it that triggers this self-destructive cascade that causes such pain and suffering—and in some cases, even death?

—⚊—

SIX WEEKS AFTER my birth, Mum could no longer hold me—the pain in her fingers had become too great. After nine months with the brakes on, her immune system was starting to return to business as usual. Cells capable of killing came back to life, and a howling wind of hormones began to blow in new directions.

As Mum's immune system returned to its normal functioning, some error triggered a chain reaction of destruction that spread through her body, year after year. Her fingers and toes became contorted beyond all recognition; complete exhaustion rendered her bedridden, and she was unable to walk. Her body slowly collapsed—she had developed rheumatoid arthritis. The cells of her immune system were confused, tricked into thinking that completely healthy parts of her body were foreign enemies. They were mutineers in her body's vital defenses.

As Christmas approached, Mum had to leave it to others to pick me up whenever I needed comfort. "It'll pass," said Dad—but uncertainty hung in the air. Mum was a doctor. Perhaps she already feared that something was seriously wrong. That the instinctive duty of care she felt for me, her newborn daughter, would be swallowed up by the darkness of a disease where our roles would become reversed. Where I would have to take care of her.

I never got a sibling. Over the course of my childhood, Mum faded away before my eyes.

Touch

I HELD MUM's hand carefully, so as not to hurt her strange, swollen fingers, as if I were handling a baby bird. We would sometimes take short walks together, sauntering through the neighborhood, but Mum didn't walk like other mothers. There was no skipping or running or games—everything happened in slow motion. These are my earliest memories.

In the 1980s, Liverpool, in northwest England, was a city deeply affected by the collapse of the labor market for industrial workers and dockers. These were bleak economic times, but sports fans were at least partly cheered by the fact that this was the golden age of Liverpool Football Club. One in every six of the city's employable inhabitants was out of work and money was a constant concern for many, but in my family it wasn't financial problems that colored our everyday activities. What I remember most is Mum's illness.

When I was around eight years old, we moved from the suburb of Woolton to a much larger house on the other side of the city, in Blundellsands. "She needs more open space," everyone said to me. In the new house, my mother sat in a chair by the big living room window, as if keeping watch. She was either there, or in bed—I hardly ever saw her anywhere else. Although she was burdened by her disease, she was always good to me. She said little—she was more of a loving presence.

My childhood centered on two things. I went to school and was a diligent student, then I came home and was a dutiful daughter. In the mornings I would enter the dark of the bedroom, where Mum would be dozing. In my hand I carried a bowl of Weetabix, the cereal sloshing around in cold milk.

If Mum was awake I would whisper "hello" before carefully setting the bowl on the bedside table. On a good day, she might give me a cautious smile. Her skin was shiny, like a balloon on the edge of bursting. Scars ran across her thighs, like millipedes; both her knees had prostheses. Her toes were pulled out into an unnatural V shape, as if they had been cracked apart. On the occasions she sat in the living room when there were other people around, I made sure to keep a close eye on her—her toes were a forbidden zone. If anything touched them, she writhed in agony.

When I got home from school, I would go straight in to see her again; the crispy bricks of Weetabix were by now reduced to a soft, sludge-like porridge. The sores in her mouth made all food seem like sandpaper, so she was often unable to eat. I would carry the tepid mixture down to the kitchen. A daily defeat.

Mum couldn't sleep alone, so on the nights my father needed a break I would lie in bed beside her. We would get up and turn her during the night, tentatively moving her frail, ever more emaciated body. One wrong move or a hand that gripped too hard and she would groan with pain.

In the half-dark of the bedroom, Mum's thin arms lay stretched out along the sides of the bed. They ended in red, swollen finger joints, her fingers permanently bent, like the neck of a swan.

MY FATHER WAS strict, and the importance of doing well at school was impressed upon me from a young age. Helping me to learn was Dad's way of showing how much he cared about me. He taught me how to read when I was three years old, and at school I became one of the best students in my class. I felt this was the only way of making Dad happy.

When I came home from school, I would usually sneak a few minutes of children's TV; as soon as I heard Dad's car come up the

driveway I would turn the TV off and make a start on my home-
work. Mum cared little for school or success—she only wanted me
to be happy. Perhaps living with an illness makes good grades and
careers seem less important than other things in life.

Our house eventually functioned like a nursing home. We had
domestic help, and relatives often visited to help out—aunts and
cousins living with us for months at a time to reduce the strain on
Dad and me. Our home life meant that I never had friends over—it
wasn't that I didn't have friends, but I had no desire to bring my
primary-school classmates home to a hospital.

I accepted the situation. Children who experience such challenges early in life often take on a lot of responsibility. I cared
about and looked out for the other children at school—to my
teachers I was probably the perfect student. A mature and con-
scientious little girl.

OUR FAMILY SITUATION changed my father. As the years passed,
he put more and more distance between himself and what was
happening at home. I remember feeling that he'd given up, and
that even more of the burden was then transferred to me.

Mum sank deeper into the darkness that surrounds all serious
illnesses. She seemed depressed. Her social life vanished—family
friends mostly stopped by to check that everything was ticking
over, not to chat about what had happened over the past week.
Her helplessness also embarrassed her. The few visitors who came
to the house were forced to go into the dark bedroom to greet her,
and she eventually tried to avoid this as much as possible. The days
became a repetitive affair, filled with pain and melancholy.

I come from a family of doctors, and since Mum was also a doctor, she understood better than most just how bad her situation

was. She was suffering from a serious case of a disease she knew would only worsen with time, and so I don't think it was long before she stopped fighting it. In the early 1980s there were few treatments available, so hope for a better future was practically nonexistent. My parents never spoke to me about these things; we rarely spoke at all. Our main focus was on getting Mum through one day at a time.

Luckily, memory is a sorting machine that generally wants what's best for us, and one of my most vivid memories of Mum is a happy one. It was our last journey together—a trip to London to meet the most famous woman in the world.

A last smile

SHE'S SO TALL, I thought as I walked across the stage toward her. Princess Diana held out her hand to me; I took it with my clammy one. "Congratulations," she said, a word she must have uttered countless times in her role as a member of the royal family.

She was elegant, as always, in a blue skirt and red buttoned jacket, her earrings oversized, shining yellow spheres. But even to a thirteen-year-old it was clear that she wasn't completely present. This Wednesday, February 10, 1993, marked two months since she and Prince Charles had announced their separation. She was in the middle of the world's most talked-about breakup.

Alongside 150 other children from all across the United Kingdom, I received the Child of Achievement Award at a prestigious ceremony held at the Queen Elizabeth II Centre in Westminster, London. The prize was awarded to children who had excelled in various areas, and not even royal relationship problems could dampen the joy and excitement felt by those of us who attended.

My dutiful life—in which I juggled being good at school with being a carer at home—had been acknowledged.

The room was full of children, parents, celebrities, and other guests. Among them, Mum sat in her wheelchair. She was wearing a red jacket and round, wobbly gold earrings. The thirteen-year battle against her illness was evident in her face—she had the characteristic moon face, a well-known side effect of years spent taking high-dose cortisone. The rest of her body was skin and bone. She was so proud that day. Her face broke into the genuine but cautious smile I had barely seen in years.

The trip to London was like a holiday—we rarely left our suburb of Liverpool. And staying in a hotel together was fantastic. Even my dad was in a good mood. To have two happy parents seemed like a miracle at the time. They saw that recognition could also be paid to people who had been dealt a poor hand in life. Maybe it gave my mother hope to know that something good had come out of it all—something that gave meaning to the meaningless pain.

Five weeks later her condition worsened, and she had to go into the hospital. We were used to this—she was continually being admitted with complications. But this time she didn't return home.

"She stayed alive so she could be at your award ceremony," said a friend of the family. Maybe she did, for all I know. And perhaps painful experiences can also give people drive. The drive to create meaning in their life's story.

Release

"ANITA, COME WITH ME, your mother is very sick." I glanced toward the door of the classroom, where a family friend was beckoning to me. My heart sank. Despite Mum's countless hospital admissions, I had never been collected from school. The day before she had been in good spirits, sitting up in the hospital bed and seemingly alert, even cheerful. I've since heard the same said of cancer patients—that their condition often seems to improve slightly just before they die.

The tiles on the floor of the hospital corridor were diamond shaped; children often look at the floor when concerned or afraid. Outside Mum's room were several familiar faces, people who had come to say their goodbyes. Some of them bowed their heads; others looked at me with teary eyes. Nobody said anything, but I understood the looks they gave me. Those looks carried silent voices that said: "We're sorry."

I took a deep breath and entered the room. It was silent. Beside the bed, nurses stood administering glucose to Mum from cotton swabs, to prevent her mouth from drying out. It was as if she was already gone.

I sat on the chair beside the bed. Her mouth was half open, her breathing heavy, as if every breath was a struggle. In retrospect, as a doctor, I know that my mother had developed an embolism in her lungs that made it difficult for her to breathe. Perhaps they decided to let nature run its course because she was so ill, choosing instead to focus on ensuring that she would feel as little pain as possible at the end.

A hoarse whisper came from her mouth: "*Pani... pani...*" The word for "water" in her native tongue—was she thirsty? Her words were difficult to interpret; perhaps merely the restlessness of a consciousness slipping away.

Suddenly I saw my dear friend Suneet in the doorway. One of the neighborhood kids, a sweet Indian boy with caramel-brown eyes, always neat and well-dressed. I smoothed down my hair and smiled shyly. What was he doing here? "Hi, Anita," he said, cautiously. He pulled up a chair, sat beside me, and placed a hand on my shoulder. "Hi," I answered. There wasn't much more to say. We were children, and death felt so grown-up.

Watching a parent die—the experience becomes permanently etched in one's memory. Everyone at the hospital that day knew it was the end. But nobody told thirteen-year-old me that Mum was about to leave forever.

I'd never thought that she might die of her disease—we were supposed to always be together, remain a family. I used to imagine future scenarios, playing them out in my mind, problems we might have to solve. What if another world war broke out? How would she get to safety if she couldn't walk? Death had never seemed an option to me until later that day, when my father and I sat in the car on the way home from the hospital.

"Do you think Mum's going to die?" I asked.

"Yes," Dad answered. He didn't cry—at least, never in front of me. But later my cousin told me that my father had cried that day.

We went into the house. *Mum's never coming home*, I thought.

I had never experienced the feeling of a happy home. Anyone who has lived with someone who is ill over an extended period of time knows that this creates a special kind of atmosphere. The constant presence of disease carries with it an aura of grief. I noticed how relaxed I became when visiting the homes of friends, which were just like homes should be. Our house had a shadow cast over it. Sometimes it was like entering someone else's house. Now the shadow had withdrawn—Mum was dying. It was a relief.

"I'll get us takeaway," said Dad. It was a kind of tradition—whenever Mum was in the hospital, we bought fish and chips from the local chip shop. For me this was synonymous with taking a break from sickness, in a home free from shadows.

—◈—

AT NINE O'CLOCK the next morning, a Saturday, the telephone rang. She was dead.

I walked down the hospital corridor at Dad's side. He came to work here every day, but this was anything but the same old everyday routine. *It must be strange for him*, I thought. He was always so controlled; we didn't rush down the corridor, there was no drama. It could have been just another ordinary day. I'd never seen a dead person before, and I was apprehensive. Dad's silence didn't help much.

Saturday mornings at the hospital were quiet. A nurse passed us and gave us a sympathetic nod. Then we were standing at the door to death itself. Dad slowly opened the door and went in. I peered hesitantly through the opening, then crept into the room. Her eyes were closed, her mouth wide open, as if she were still trying to breathe. She didn't look dead. Were they sure? I thought I heard sounds coming from deep within her. "Yes, she's dead," said Dad. Sounds were normal. Mum was gone.

"Feel how soft her hands are," said Dad, stroking and squeezing her fingers. He was right—her hands were soft. I thought that was a nice thing to say. All the pain was gone. Dad leaned toward her face and touched her cheek. "I'll look after Anita," he said.

I wondered how things would be from now on. We had never had a normal life, we had always been different—life's daily routines had always centered on Mum. I thought of all the times I'd slept in the bed beside her at night. How that was all over now.

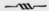

AT HOME A few days later, an open casket lay in the large, sun-filled hall. Mum was dressed in a beautiful pink sari—one of her favorites. The extra rouge and lipstick made her look a little strange, but she looked pretty. I glanced down at my new black shoes; they had small heels. For the first time, I felt like a grown-up.

The house was full of Indian friends and a number of my father's colleagues from the hospital. It was good to feel the warmth of the people who were there to support us. The room was full of low voices and compassion. An unfamiliar atmosphere for a family isolated by illness.

I was unable to feel sad—I'd already processed my grief over several years. Instead, I felt an overwhelming sense of relief. No more suffering for Mum. No more suffering for us. I was unable to put on any kind of act, and so tried to remain in the background. Taking my place among the large group of mourners didn't come naturally to me—I was already looking ahead, toward a new chapter in my life. A chapter free from illness.

In a quiet moment, I went across to the hall bookshelf. With my mother as the only witness, I took down volume R of the *Encyclopaedia Britannica*, its brown cover smelling of leather. I sat down, opened the book, and turned the pages until I found the entry for rheumatoid arthritis. And then I began to read.

A sense of meaning began to seep into me as my eyes worked their way through the words. Joints, pain, genes, inflammation, T cells. All that had gone on in Mum's body; an entire world I knew nothing about. *Why does it happen?* All the unanswered questions sparked off new trains of thought, which curiously seemed to bring me closer to Mum. In the background I heard low voices from the hall, but they didn't reach me. This was my world alone.

My first taste of discovery. A moment I constantly return to— the start of my journey into the mysteries of the immune system. Right then, I decided that I would become a researcher. All questions have an answer. It's simply about looking in the right place.

—⚏—

THOSE FIRST YEARS after Mum's death were a chaotic mix of teenage rebellion and turmoil; a reaction to all that needed to come out, an overcompensation for an isolated childhood. I went from being a straight-A student to a rebel who ended up with Ds and Fs. But at a certain point, I ran out of things to lash out at. I left home at seventeen, returned to my studies, and ended up in the newspaper as one of the students with the best exam results in England.

I had an aim in sight: medical school. There, I became completely obsessed with the body's defenses—the immune system. The very same cells that had stolen my mother's life.

2

THE MASTER
AND A CLUE

*"The body's failure to recognize itself,
its capacity to treat itself as foreign, seems
both sinister and bizarre."*
WARWICK ANDERSON AND IAN R. MACKAY,
INTOLERANT BODIES, 2014

"AREN'T YOU TIRED of us yet?"
Roger Bucknall laughed when he saw me. The experienced doctor was no longer surprised at the fact that I continually turned up in the rheumatology department of the Royal Liverpool University Hospital. In the corridor, doctors hurried past me, on their way to see patients with swollen fingers, stiff backs, and silent spasms of pain in their faces. The beeping of pagers accompanied the squeaking of shoes on the linoleum floor. This was the hospital where my mum had worked twenty-three years earlier. Now I was here, undertaking my practical training as a medical student.

"Tired of you? No! This is where I belong."

Most of the other medical students wanted to gain experience in as many fields as possible—neurology, cardiology, gastroenterology, and so on. But I was interested in just one thing. The encyclopedia I had read on the day of Mum's funeral had said that rheumatoid arthritis was a rheumatological disease. So I chose rheumatology as my selected area of study—not once, but every time I had the option to choose.

A rheumatologist works with diseases that affect the muscles, joints, and tendons, that result in inflammation and wear. Many patients with autoimmune diseases ended up in the rheumatology department. Dr. Bucknall had been there for years and seen pretty much all there was to see. He was a well-dressed man who maintained eye contact when he spoke to you, and although he wasn't the kind of person who smiled all the time, he had a good, very dry—and very British—sense of humor.

He started work every day at eight o'clock in the morning, with patients moving in and out of his office at a rapid tempo. Books, scientific papers, and other documents were stacked as high as skyscrapers in there—it was a veritable Manhattan of paper. He loved rheumatology and was probably intrigued by the single-minded student who repeatedly returned to work with him. We developed a close working relationship, which eventually became a friendship.

I quickly found that I could ask Dr. Bucknall about anything. If he didn't know the answer to my question, he always made sure to find me someone who did. This wasn't always successful, however. Because I'd repeatedly asked about what happened to the immune system in cases of rheumatoid arthritis, Bucknall called one of his colleagues, a professor of immunology. He described me as a talented student, and I was granted an audience with the esteemed professor in his office so that I could ask him a few questions. This was so early on in our course that we hadn't yet been given a single immunology lecture.

The professor showed me into his office; I took a seat in the chair in front of his desk. He looked at me, his expression indicating that it was now up to me to steer the conversation.

"Could you tell me about theta cells?" I asked, tightening my grip on my pen, ready to make notes. His features twisted into an almost pained expression that I'll never forget. Because the immune system contains no such thing as theta cells. I'd misunderstood some of the literature I'd read, and had now asked a completely ridiculous question.

"Do you mean T cells?" asked the professor with a sigh. I squirmed in my chair and nodded cautiously, and not long afterward he found an excuse to get me out of his office. He had no interest in spending his valuable time on lackadaisical students.

The experience was highly embarrassing, not least because Bucknall had arranged the meeting and spoken so highly of me. In the British medical world professors are regarded with the greatest respect. Students are seen, but rarely heard. It was special to be given the chance to meet with a professor for a private lesson, and therefore even more embarrassing to make such a spectacular mistake.

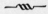

STUDENTS OFTEN ACCOMPANIED the professors on their rounds, standing around each patient's bed as the professor ran the show. In England, the doctors are always well dressed: the men in a shirt and tie, the women in smart trousers and heeled shoes. Some of the professors were notoriously strict. One story circulating among us told of a student who hadn't taken the time to shave that morning. During the rounds, with the patient in the bed and the other students gathered around, the professor had looked at the unlucky student in dismay. Then he took a coin from his pocket, threw it at the poor guy, and said: "Buy yourself a razor, would you please?"

But Roger Bucknall was different. He listened with interest to all the questions I asked as a young and naive student. If he had an interesting patient, he would fetch me and tell me there was someone I should meet. Through my first enthusiastic encounters with the world of autoimmunity, he became my mentor.

All these diseases, and so few answers. I met a boy of just fifteen, so emaciated that I wondered whether he would survive. He should have been playing football or running after girls, but instead he was bedridden in the hospital with juvenile idiopathic arthritis. On other days I would meet women with a red, butterfly-shaped rash spreading from the bridge of their nose and out across their cheeks—typical of patients with lupus, a disease that is infamously difficult to diagnose. Joint pain, mouth ulcers, hair loss, sensitivity to light, fatigue, chest pains, and occasionally even psychosis: not one of the body's organs is safe from lupus, a beast that switches back and forth between hibernation mode and wild rage.

I saw patients with the whitish, scaly scabs characteristic of a disease that affects around 2 percent of us. In some patients this itchy rash spreads across large areas of the back, while in others there are only small patches around the eyes. Psoriasis is a red, irritating stress alarm that sounds on and off throughout patients' lives—but they can live with it. Unfortunately, the same cannot be said for the middle-aged women with small sores that appear on their fingertips, like tiny potholes; the thick, shiny skin that pulls tight like a fishing net, making it difficult to use the hands. These women have systemic sclerosis, in which there is thickened connective tissue in the skin and injuries to the small blood vessels, which can progress to the internal organs. Doctors try to put the brakes on the immune system, but in the end the patient's heart, lungs, or kidneys often fail, and this can be fatal.

Meeting these patients was like rediscovering my mum. It was therapeutic. I walked home from the clinic every day with the sense that I was doing something right. But at the same time, I saw how much suffering these patients endured. And how little hope they had to cling to.

"Then it spreads throughout the entire body…"

AN AUTOIMMUNE REACTION can occur at any time; none of the body's organs or systems are safe from possible attack. These reactions result in a broad range of diseases with vastly different symptoms. There are probably over a hundred diseases in which autoimmunity plays an important role, and this number continues to grow as researchers make new discoveries.

I was most interested in the disease my mum had suffered from. Around one in every hundred people will develop rheumatoid arthritis—it's one of the most common autoimmune diseases we know of. In some patients the joints are completely destroyed and deformed into the disease's characteristic appearance.

Portrayals of such deformed joints enable us to trace the disease through both art and literature. When the Dutch artist Rubens painted *The Three Graces* in 1635, it was hardly his poor handiwork that resulted in the fingers of one of the women in the painting stretching out at an unnatural angle—something that would be impossible for a healthy hand to achieve. Several of Rubens's paintings feature hands with classic symptoms of rheumatoid arthritis, and medical historians have speculated that the world-renowned painter may have suffered from the disease himself. This information has informed the debate about whether this is a disease that has arisen during the modern age, or whether it can be traced further back through history.

Hippocrates, the father of clinical medicine, is among those who described symptoms reminiscent of the disease over two thousand years ago. According to the Greek philosopher, the symptoms appeared in patients around the age of thirty-five. In the same period, similar descriptions were also circulating in the country of my ancestors. Charaka, the "Indian Hippocrates," wrote about patients who experienced pain, stiffness, and shrinkage in the joints. "It first affects the hands and feet, then it spreads throughout the entire body," wrote Charaka. He also mentioned the characteristic swelling that can occur with rheumatoid arthritis, which presents as pea-sized lumps beneath the skin. According to Charaka, these were like "bags full of air, and movements involving bending and stretching cause pain."

Historians credit the French surgeon Augustin Jacob Landré-Beauvais with providing the first certain description of rheumatoid arthritis, in a doctoral thesis in the year 1800. At the Salpêtrière Hospital in Paris, he monitored nine patients suffering from the classic symptoms. Most rheumatic diseases were classified under the umbrella term "rheumatism" at the time, but Landré-Beauvais believed that the nine patients he was monitoring were distinct. He described a chronic disease that affected several joints, led to a poor state of general health, and primarily affected women. Over fifty years later, the disease was given the name medical professionals use to describe it to this day: rheumatoid arthritis.

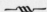

IN RECENT DECADES we have developed increasingly effective treatments for rheumatoid arthritis, but no cure. Every tenth patient suffers such a severe case of the disease that they may become markedly disabled. A disease's perceived severity is often based on how lethal it is—we fear cancer and heart disease because these are diseases so closely associated with death. But an increasing number of patients also survive these diseases, and live good lives for many years afterward. It's easy to think that rheumatoid arthritis is less serious—because surely you can't die from it, right?

But the truth is that rheumatoid arthritis can also affect the internal organs. On average, patients with rheumatoid arthritis live lives that are several years shorter than those of healthy individuals. Some might die of heart disease, but the guilty party here is still the rheumatoid arthritis, having worn down the body over many years. The same is true for a number of other auto-immune diseases. They are among the leading causes of death in the world, particularly for young and middle-aged women. My mother was just fifty-one years old when she became part of these bleak statistics.

Now I was meeting patients in the hospital where my mother had once worked, back when she became pregnant with me. Where she probably spent time thinking about her future, about family life in the new country to which she was slowly becoming accustomed. But all that would remain a dream.

Hormone histories

ONE OF MY best friends in Liverpool was born on the same day as me—and even at the same hospital. And as if that wasn't enough, her mum had rheumatoid arthritis, too. Like Mum, my friend's mother had developed the disease right after giving birth. It was hard to believe that this was a coincidence, and as a medical student I was finally in a position to look for answers. I thoroughly interrogated every patient I encountered in the rheumatology department. When did you first experience the symptoms? Have you been pregnant? What happened during your pregnancy? What happened after you gave birth?

My research career was already underway during my time as a medical student. I didn't just want to examine and treat my patients—I wanted to trace a path back to the source of the disease. I've always been like this. As a child I would spend hours perfecting my school assignments, constantly on the lookout for ingenious solutions. I'd always wanted to be a researcher, even back then. I now saw that it was possible to follow my dream.

Might pregnancy tell us something important about what causes rheumatoid arthritis and other autoimmune diseases? If so, it must have something to do with the fact that the body changes when a woman becomes pregnant. Of course the body changes—just look at the hormones, which are greatly affected by pregnancy. Hormones carry messages around the body, stage-directing everything from stress and the conversion of energy to growth and reproduction. It was therefore striking to hear case histories that connected the disease to hormonal changes. The patients clearly remembered when their lives had changed, and I listened to them with ever-increasing interest.

"I experienced the first symptoms a few weeks after giving birth."

"It started around the time I entered menopause."

"I noticed it right after I started taking hormone-suppressing medicines."

I started to ask myself what the connection might be between hormonal changes and the start of the disease. Later, I completed a survey of eighty-three women with rheumatoid arthritis. In over half of the women, the disease arose directly after pregnancy or during menopause—that is, in a period of significant changes in the body's production of sex hormones. Might sex hormones be the key?

Some research had been done into hormones and rheumatoid arthritis, but with regard to what my patients were telling me, there was astoundingly little. I threw myself into reading the available reports, and my suspicions were soon confirmed. Many women became ill just after giving birth. The bodily changes that occur in connection with having a child seemed to be able to trigger the disease. Another interesting piece of information was that in most cases, the condition of women already suffering from rheumatoid arthritis improved significantly during pregnancy. Something suppressed the disease for nine months, but after birth the opposite was true—the women experienced an intense worsening of their symptoms. Nobody knew for sure why this happened. An unknown factor obviously played a role, and it was this unknown factor I wanted to identify.

But at the same time, something happened that would have far-reaching consequences for the rest of my life and career. One morning, I met Robin.

A Norwegian crosses my path

"HI, I'VE BEEN looking for you," said the young guy standing in front of me. His endearing accent indicated that he wasn't British. *Oh you have, have you?* I thought. *Well, I haven't been looking for you.* But before I could say anything, he continued: "I'm your mentor."

So this is Robin, I thought. On my first day at medical school I'd found his name written beside mine on the noticeboard. Robin was in the year above me and was supposed to act as a kind of one-man welcome committee. I'd decided I had no use for a mentor and so hadn't bothered to turn up at the designated place where the mentors were supposed to meet with the new students. But now he'd found me anyway. I wondered whether I should just brush him off, tell him I wasn't interested. But there was something about the guy. He was weird and funny in a way that I could relate to. So I politely introduced myself.

"It would be nice to have a chat," he continued. I hesitated, hardly enthusiastic. "Come on, I insist," he said, smiling.

He seemed like the serious type, and to get through the small talk we'd need to loosen up a little. It was the start of the semester, with endless student parties and events that lasted from late in the evening into the early hours. This would be my one morning indulgence as a first-year student, I decided, as I never took part in any of the other festivities.

"Okay, maybe we should go to the pub," I said, trying to act cool and not in the slightest bit fazed by the fact that it was still early in the morning. Robin nodded, satisfied, and took me to the nearest watering hole. There, he threw his jacket over the back of a chair and glanced at the bar. "What would you like?"

"Vodka and coke?" I said cheekily as I took a seat on the opposite side of the table. He raised his eyebrows almost imperceptibly, possibly wondering who on earth he'd been paired up with. But he brought the drinks to the table, and that's how I got to know Robin from Porsgrunn, Norway.

We started to spend more and more time together. Robin would dish up Norwegian salmon dinners and we'd take weekend trips away all across the United Kingdom. In the year in which he could have taken his date to see the romantic *Notting Hill* at the movies, he instead chose the horror film *The Blair Witch Project*.

After a few months Robin invited me to celebrate Christmas and New Year's with him in Norway. I gladly accepted, and arrived in Norway in December wearing high heels. The fact that there might be snow on the ground hadn't even occurred to me, but cold feet didn't stop me falling head over heels for the charming country with its colorful houses. There was something unpretentious about the Norwegian people, who refused to be subdued by freezing temperatures and icy roads. I was used to spending my holidays in noisy, smelly, hot and humid India. Norway had a wonderful sense of calm about it. To me, Norway was just as exotic as India might seem to Norwegians. I felt immediately safe and grounded in the country—despite the high heels.

A few months later, Robin and I got engaged in secret. It felt right to do it that way, and we eloped in Svalbard just a short time later. My father didn't take the news particularly well—the fact that I had married in secret without the family's blessing was shameful to him. He had changed in the years following Mum's death, and we'd gradually grown apart. After I married Robin, any contact we'd had was severed completely.

—⁓—

DURING MY MEDICAL training at the hospital in Liverpool I'd listened to story after story from women who had developed rheumatoid arthritis right after giving birth. The same thing had happened to my mum. Then I became pregnant. Should I be nervous that the same disease might be lying dormant within me? Was it hiding there, biding its time, just waiting for an opportunity to break free?

3

NATURE VERSUS NURTURE

"Autoimmune diseases appear to be a mismatch between genes and the environment."
DAVID HAFLER, CHAIRMAN OF THE DEPARTMENT OF NEUROLOGY AT YALE SCHOOL OF MEDICINE, TO THE *WASHINGTON POST* IN 2016

K ANPUR IS A city of several million inhabitants in the north of India, known for its production of high-quality leather—an industry that puts the city toward the top of the list of the most polluted places in the country. Every morning the sun's rays struggle to penetrate a blanket of smog. This is where my mum grew up.

When I was small, we would travel to Kanpur every summer to visit family. I loved to travel. The tiny boxes of airplane food; the attentive cabin crew, eager to look after a precocious little girl. Over the years I had become familiar with Heathrow Airport in London, where I would push Mum in her wheelchair through the departure hall and to the gate.

On her last trips to India Mum mainly stayed inside, lying in bed in a darkened room because she was so ill. But it was still a relief for her to arrive in Kanpur, because there she was no longer my burden to carry. There were sisters, brothers, cousins, and her mother—an entire family who could take responsibility for her. For a few idyllic weeks I could simply be a child.

We stayed in a garage-like house in which the doors were holes cut out in the wall. Guava trees grew in the backyard, and monkeys binged on the red and yellow fruits. In the corner was a plastic tank filled with water, a jug lapping at its surface. This was the shower. Here, giggling children might encounter their grandmother, who, somewhat less self-conscious than the rest of us, washed with nothing but a small piece of cloth around her waist. In the mornings we formed a curious audience for the milkman, who sat outside the door milking the cow he'd brought with him. A guarantee that the milk hadn't been diluted with water.

Our journeys to India were like opening the door to a wardrobe and passing through it into a completely new world. Everything was different. The toilets were holes in the ground with the shapes of footprints on either side to indicate where you should squat. Once, when I was visiting the local school, a snake peeked up out of the toilet hole—an event I enthusiastically told the teacher about. Not long afterward they sent in a man decked out in full Ghostbusters equipment to get rid of it. To think I could have spent my last moments going to the toilet!

My genes are of course inherited from my Indian parents—they can be traced back thousands of years, and through the process of evolution have developed in accordance with the surrounding environment. The descriptions of my childhood holidays illustrate how an Indian child grows up in a completely different environment than a British one. Mum grew up in India, while I grew up in England. And because of this, I actually have an increased risk of rheumatoid arthritis compared to my mum. But why?

The disease code

EVERY CELL OF our body contains our genetic material—our DNA—twisted together into highly compact packages we call chromosomes. This is where we find the genes, the instruction manual for the world's most complicated construction set: the human body. If we were to stretch out all the DNA in the body's several thousand billion cells, we'd create a line estimated to be twice the diameter of our solar system.

In the year 2000, researchers from the international Human Genome Project presented the result of a decade of work costing US$3 billion. For the first time, we were able to see the total DNA content of a cell—what we call the human genome. The recipe for a person was no longer a secret; billions of codes had fallen into place. But some were disappointed to learn that the most dominant being on earth—the human—consists of no more than around twenty thousand functional genes. This is around the same number as in a millimeter-long roundworm. The functional genes comprise less than 2 percent of the human genome. The rest is genomic dark matter we still know very little about.

Our genes determine how susceptible we are to developing diseases. It's well known that most diseases are hereditary, and some more so than others. So just how hereditary are autoimmune diseases? Nature has provided us with the ideal experiment to investigate heredity: identical twins. Identical twins have identical DNA. If autoimmune diseases were 100 percent hereditary, then if one of the twins developed a disease, the other would too. But this is far from the case—on average, there is around a 30 percent chance that the second twin will develop the same disease. This genetic risk varies depending on the autoimmune disease.

Because my mum had rheumatoid arthritis, my risk of developing the disease is around three times greater than that of others.

This sounds like a lot, but since the risk is so low to start with, it means that my chances of becoming ill are still small. Let's say that one person in every hundred will develop rheumatoid arthritis. A risk three times this still only means that three people in every hundred will develop rheumatoid arthritis. In other words, the chance of not getting the disease is much greater.

Which is to say: my mum wasn't born destined to become ill. Many people live with a genetic predisposition for rheumatoid arthritis, but only a few ever develop the disease. Something has to trigger it, and this is where the environment comes into play. Although I've inherited my genes from my Indian mum and dad, I've grown up in England—in an environment that makes me more susceptible to most autoimmune diseases, including rheumatoid arthritis.

A decisive childhood

RESEARCH INTO AUTOIMMUNE diseases doesn't have a very long history. Only in the 1950s did researchers discover that the body was able to attack itself, and over subsequent decades they found out that this wasn't an uncommon phenomenon. But it took a long time before anyone started to count the number of patients. Until the 1990s, we knew little about how many people suffer from autoimmune diseases, who they are, and where they live.

When researchers started this kind of epidemiological research, it became apparent that where you live is a decisive factor in your risk of becoming ill. For example, we now know that in Western Europe around six women in every thousand have rheumatoid arthritis. In the area my parents come from, this figure is only two to three women in every thousand. Those who are born and grow up in parts of Asia and Africa are less likely to develop autoimmune diseases than people from Western countries. It's easy to think that this is solely down to genes, but it's not that simple.

In recent decades, people have had far greater opportunities to cross borders and move between different parts of the world. This significant growth in emigration and immigration has made it possible to study how the environment in which we grow up affects our chances of developing various diseases. And the results of such studies are striking.

Let's take a look at the autoimmune disease multiple sclerosis (MS). This is a disease in which the cells of the immune system attack the insulation surrounding the body's neural pathways. It's as if someone sends a horde of rats into the nervous system to chew on each and every live cable they can find. Norway is one of the countries in the world in which inhabitants have the greatest risk of developing MS.

In the 1970s, a large group of immigrants from Pakistan arrived in Norway, settling there to work and bring up their families and integrating into Norwegian society. Generally, people from Pakistan have a lower risk of developing MS than people from Norway. But what happened after they moved to this new country?

It turned out that the children of the Pakistani immigrants had a risk of developing MS that was three times greater than that of their parents who had moved to Norway as adults. That is, it wasn't only their genes that influenced their risk of developing the disease. "The sharp increase in prevalence in immigrants seen in one generation suggests strong environmental factors affecting the MS risk in Norway," concluded the researchers behind the study. Something about the Norwegian environment or lifestyle means that people who grow up in Norway have a greater chance of developing MS as adults, and the same trend can be seen for a number of other autoimmune diseases.

People who live in England also have a high risk of developing diseases such as MS and rheumatoid arthritis—higher than in India. When my mum and dad moved to England and had me, the same thing that happened to the Pakistani immigrants in Norway happened within our family: my chances of developing rheumatoid arthritis increased. Our genes are responsible for around half the risk of developing rheumatoid arthritis, while environmental factors stand for the rest. It is only when predisposed genes encounter the right triggers that we become ill.

Environmental factors can include diet, infections, sunlight, chemicals, medications, hormonelike substances, pollution, and countless other things—in short, everything in the environment around us and the culture in which we live affects the body. Speculation regarding which environmental factors actually play a role in triggering autoimmune diseases extends far and wide, but the truth is that we know very little about this. One of the most well-known environmental factors, however, is smoking. You have a far greater chance of developing rheumatoid arthritis if you smoke—but only if you also have a genetic predisposition for the disease. The interplay between nature and nurture determines whether or not you will become ill.

I WASN'T AFRAID that I would develop rheumatoid arthritis when I became pregnant as a medical student—the chances were still very low. I saw my pregnancy as a perfect opportunity to dig deep into the effects of this bodily upheaval on my patients. This was, after all, what I was interested in.

More and more patients came through the doors of the rheumatology department of the hospital in Liverpool and told me about how pregnancy had changed their lives in more ways than one. What fascinated me most was the women already suffering from rheumatoid arthritis when they became pregnant. Many of them enthusiastically told me about how dramatically their condition had improved over those nine months. *Wow*, I thought. Pregnancy seemed to be an effective medicine against rheumatoid arthritis. Completely natural and without side effects.

But at the same time doubt kept jabbing me in the shoulder, because the connection seemed so obvious. Why were so few researchers interested in this? Surely others must have wondered about the same thing? That was when I came across the story of a medical miracle.

4

A DANCE
OUT OF THE
WHEELCHAIR

*"The thought occurred: Instead of being
relentlessly progressive, this disease, rheumatoid
arthritis, may be potentially reversible, more so
than we have believed, perhaps rapidly so."*
PHILIP S. HENCH, IN HIS NOBEL LECTURE, 1950

PHILIP HENCH WORKED at the Mayo Clinic in the United
States in the 1920s. Here, the young doctor met with
patients suffering from rheumatoid arthritis, who told him
the same stories I myself heard every day. Hench's patients said
that they felt better while pregnant but then experienced a severe
relapse after giving birth. Hench noted a similar improvement in
patients with jaundice and those who were fasting. He wondered
whether the body, under certain circumstances, produced a substance that alleviated rheumatoid arthritis. And if so, might it be
possible to find a medicine against the terrible disease—perhaps
even a cure? This became the start of Hench's long search for what
he called substance X.

At the time, there was no treatment to offer patients suffering from rheumatoid arthritis. They were simply given hot baths—this was all that could be done for them. Crippled, aching bodies suffered in their hospital beds, the equivalent of today's terminal cancer patients. Hench was faced with this hopelessness every single day, and it must have been a huge motivating force. Because just imagine if a cure was within reach. "It would be gratifying if one were able to repeat nature's miracle," wrote Hench of his search for substance X. He gave his patients ox bile and bile salts; he tried blood transfusions using the blood of a patient with jaundice in an attempt to recreate the palliative effect. It was an endless cycle of trial and error in the hope of finding substance X. Since such vastly different things as pregnancy and jaundice improved his patients' conditions, Hench believed substance X must be a substance the body produced for various reasons. Hench thought it might be a hormone, and so he fairly quickly set his sights on the adrenal glands.

The hormones produced by the adrenal glands had not yet been discovered, but researchers knew that they must exist. Finding them would be a race toward groundbreaking discoveries, with all the honor and esteem this would afford. During the Second World War, rumors were circulating about German pilots, who were said to be able to fly up to forty thousand feet because they were injected with a substance extracted from the adrenal glands—a kind of superserum. American spies reported that the Germans were sending submarines to Argentina to purchase huge numbers of adrenal glands from cattle in order to mass-produce the substance. The rumors were hardly true, but they did result in intensified efforts to find out more about these fabled hormones.

The history of research is full of strokes of luck, and Hench was lucky enough to be working at the same hospital as the chemist

Edward Kendall. Kendall was among the most eminent researchers working on the adrenal glands, and he and Hench began to
collaborate. In the early 1940s, after years of cooking up various
concoctions in the laboratory, the pair believed that they had
the answer. Producing sufficient amounts of the substance was
a laborious task that required vast quantities of adrenal glands
from animals. The Second World War certainly didn't make it any
easier to be a researcher, and so Hench was forced to wait before
he could finally complete the experiment he had been working
toward for over a decade—to test substance X on his patients.

Pharmaceutical company Merck produced the substance, but
doing so was a complex process, and they were starting to lose
patience with the blasted hormone—it had cost them huge sums
of money and brought them little in return. Indeed, the rumors
about the German superpilots had turned out to be absolute non-
sense. Perhaps it was time to bring the entire hormone production
process to a close. In 1948, only a measly nine grams remained
of what Hench believed to be the magical substance X. In a last
attempt to find a use for the hormone, Merck gave it away to
selected groups of researchers. Hench was given five grams.

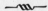

I CAN JUST imagine his nervous smile. He'd been working
toward this moment for his entire career, and now he had five
valuable grams in his hand. Failure was not an option, because
Merck wasn't interested in producing any more. Hench needed
indisputable evidence that substance X was worthy of further
investigation. His selected test patient was Mrs. Gardner, a twenty-
nine-year-old woman with severe rheumatoid arthritis. She trun-
dled around the hospital corridors in a wheelchair, determinedly
refusing to leave the clinic until someone could give her some kind

of hope. Hench decided that at the very least, they shouldn't risk administering a dose that was too low.

Over the course of four days, Hench gave Mrs. Gardner 100 milligrams a day of what we now know as cortisone. Today, a usual dose is 7.5 milligrams. On the fourth day, Mrs. Gardner set aside her wheelchair, strolled out of the hospital, and went shopping. Hench's subsequent trials were no less spectacular—patients who had previously lain immobile, their limbs like twisted branches, now danced around their beds.

When Hench presented his results for the first time, in April 1949, twenty years had passed since he had first had the idea about substance X. He was a brilliant speaker and described the drama's last act to a packed auditorium. On the screen behind him, he showed film footage of a patient tiptoeing out of a wheelchair after just four days of cortisone treatment. The *New York Times* described it as a modern miracle. Soon, patients were hammering at the doors of doctors' offices all across the country in the hope of obtaining just a few milligrams of the new wonder drug.

The attentive doctor

WHAT HAD HENCH discovered after years of trial and error? He'd ended up in the hormone system that kicks in when the body is subjected to stress, such as physical activity, mental stress, or acute illness. These hormones are also a part of the fight-or-flight response. They prepare the body to handle danger—if you were to step on a viper, for example, or to break your arm. The hormones therefore regulate vital functions, such as energy production and our defenses, in order to give the body the best possible chance of survival.

Hench and Kendall discovered one of the most important hormones in this system—cortisol. In the event of acute stressors, this hormone ensures that the energy-intensive immune system calms down, so that energy can be used for other purposes. Cortisone is simply a chemical version of the hormone cortisol. Administering large doses of cortisone proved to have a powerful anti-inflammatory effect.

However, doctors quickly understood that cortisone was no wonder cure that would put out the fire for good—it only dampened the flames. The huge doses were not sustainable, because serious side effects appeared fairly rapidly: a greater risk of serious infection, diabetes, high blood pressure, brittle bones, mental changes, and the characteristic moon face, in which the face swells and becomes rounder because the distribution of the body's fat begins to change. The use of cortisone was therefore moderated significantly over the following years.

Nonetheless, this was the start of a new era in the treatment of serious inflammation and autoimmune diseases. As a student in the rheumatology department of the hospital in Liverpool, I too saw how extremely ill patients obtained dramatic relief from short-term, high-dosage treatments, while others were dependent on long-term treatment with low doses of cortisone in order to function. To date, cortisone is one of the most important medications we have. Every day, more and more people can thank Philip Hench that they are alive.

Hench was awarded the Nobel Prize in Medicine in 1950, and in his acceptance speech he expressed optimism for the future. He believed new knowledge about the alleviating effects of pregnancy on rheumatoid arthritis would soon lead to even better treatments. But over the seventy years following the cortisone revolution, few significant advances were made in research on hormones and rheumatoid arthritis.

We now know that throughout pregnancy, the amount of cortisol in the body gradually increases. As the birth draws near, pregnant women have two to three times more cortisol in their bodies than usual. After birth, this level drops again. These fluctuations in cortisol are part of the reason why women with rheumatoid arthritis get better during pregnancy, but they don't explain why the disease can arise directly after birth.

I have great admiration for Hench—a doctor who took his patients' stories seriously. It was their accounts that eventually led him to his groundbreaking discovery. The suffering he observed every day was the driving force that kept him motivated for over twenty years. There was certainly no guarantee that he would succeed—his research was like looking through oysters to find a pearl. Even after a lifetime of searching, few have the privilege of ever finding one.

I was sure that Hench was on the right track. Hormones must be part of the key to better understanding rheumatoid arthritis. Just like Hench, I was spurred on by the desire to help ease my patients' suffering—a desire to provide the relief my mum was never given. I now had an idea of where I should start my search. Maybe we needed to shift our focus from the stress hormones in the adrenal glands to the system that keeps the human race alive. Might the answer be found in the sex hormones?

The competition

IF THE SEX hormones played a crucial role in rheumatoid arthritis, then which of them was the most important? Every day I walked through the corridors of the rheumatology department, the question like an irritating itch I couldn't scratch. In my free time I would sit in the library digging up research papers, then return to the hospital and ask Dr. Bucknall to rack his brains to find answers to all my questions.

One day, as I rushed through the swinging doors below the blue sign of the Duncan Building at the university, I suddenly stopped in front of the noticeboard in reception. This was usually full of uninteresting messages, but now a colorful poster announced a competition. A research competition in rheumatology for medical students.

When I got back to the hospital I went straight to Dr. Bucknall. "Can I take part in the competition?" I asked. He nodded encouragingly, as he always did. Over the past year, I'd already spent much of my free time plowing through research into hormones and rheumatoid arthritis. I saw only one way of getting closer to answering all the questions I had. I would have to go through all the hormones and survey how they affected the immune system.

But beneath the surface, doubt gnawed away at me. Did I have the ability to come up with original ideas and conduct research in competition with others? Did I have the requisite skills to become a scientist? I was just twenty-two years old and a student. The competition was an opportunity to convince myself that I had what it took to succeed.

THE MOST IMPORTANT sex hormone for men is testosterone; for women it is estrogen. In men, testosterone is produced in the testicles, while in women estrogen is produced in the ovaries. It is these two hormones that determine whether the body will develop in a masculine or feminine direction. If you give testosterone to women, they will develop increased muscle mass and exhibit increased hair growth.

It was first and foremost estrogen that captured my interest. The amount of estrogen increases during pregnancy, the period in which my patients told me they felt better. After women give birth, their estrogen level decreases, as it does during menopause. It is in precisely these periods that rheumatoid arthritis often first appears. Several patients also told me that they had developed rheumatoid arthritis after they started taking medicines that suppress the production of estrogen. Women with breast cancer are often given such medications as part of their treatment.

At the same time, I was also starting to take an interest in one of the most common genetic diseases we know of—Turner syndrome. This is a congenital disease that only affects girls, at the rate of about 1 in 2,500. These girls are missing one of the sex chromosomes, which contain our genetic material. Normally we have two sex chromosomes, where the x chromosome is female and the y chromosome is male. Typically, if you are a woman, you have xx, or two x chromosomes, and if you are a man, you have xy. It is the y chromosome that makes men male.

Girls with Turner syndrome are missing one of their two x chromosomes, which among other things leads to a lack of estrogen. Several studies have shown that these girls have a greater chance of developing autoimmune diseases as they get older. This was yet another clue that hinted at a connection between estrogen and autoimmunity. At this point, I therefore thought that estrogen might be the key hormone.

Many hormones communicate with the immune system, and I had to look at them in context. I examined the research literature to find out what we actually knew. The spiderweb of molecules and connections grew. Over the next few weeks, I systematized the network of a number of hormones and how they affected the immune system. Surprisingly, nobody had ever done this before.

The day finally came when I presented my findings to the competition jury. Before me in the lecture hall sat a number of renowned professors of medicine, their scrutinizing gazes all turned on me. I presented my complex survey, and to my astonishment I won the competition. The £250 in prize money would of course come in handy for a poor student, but most importantly, winning the competition boosted my self-confidence.

Maybe I really did have it in me—the ability to be a researcher.

The decision

I LET MY lullaby dwindle to a low hum. In the crib, our one-year-old daughter was just drifting off to sleep. Outside the old factory windows I caught a glimpse of the pleasant dusk light. My thoughts had been churning around and around in my head ever since I'd won the student competition. I wanted to do more.

Through the bars of the crib I could hear that my daughter had fallen asleep. I got up, stroked a hand over her head, and went out into the living room. Robin and I were renting a lovely apartment in Wapping Dock, an exclusive brick building beside the port in Liverpool, although the apartment itself didn't reflect the building's beautiful facade—we had garden chairs around the dinner table and the plastic trays of microwave dinners filled the trash can. I used to say that we had the nicest apartment of all the students we knew, though our decor wasn't exactly something out of the pages of an interior design magazine. But we didn't care what anyone else might think.

Robin was in bed; I went into the bedroom and climbed in beside him. "What's on your mind?" he asked. My churning thoughts were clearly evident.

"I ought to keep going with this," I said. "Ever since the competition I've been thinking that someone has to investigate how the various hormones affect the immune system in rheumatoid arthritis. It must be possible to find out whether some are more important than others."

Robin sat up in bed, animated, immediately throwing out ideas. His enthusiasm was infectious. He took my musings seriously.

"It's an ingenious idea," he said, joking that if exciting results came from it, he'd tell everyone that it had actually been his suggestion.

Of course there were stumbling blocks. Even back then I suspected such a project would be a career killer. Researching hormones and rheumatoid arthritis didn't bring high status in the medical world. Apart from my rebellious period as a teenager, I'd always been a high achiever. I'd imagined a future filled with success; an advancing career. Was I really going to take this shot in the dark? It would be like searching for a needle in a haystack—the chance of success was small.

"But if it's your dream, you have to follow it," said Robin. "I know you can do it."

It felt like madness to start work on an extensive research project halfway through my studies, but the gaping hole in our knowledge at the intersection between hormones and the cells of the immune system bothered me immensely. I couldn't stop thinking about it. Robin's support was the final push I needed.

"Then I suppose it'll have to be a PhD," I said, smiling coyly to lessen the seriousness of what I'd just said. But I knew there and then that I meant it.

So this is where it starts, I thought. Someone had to close the gap in knowledge—or at least try to. I wanted to know whether there was a direct connection between my birth and my mum's illness. But would anyone be willing to take a chance on me and my ideas?

5

THE LONELY RESEARCHER

*"If you're not prepared to be wrong,
you'll never come up with anything original."*
SIR KEN ROBINSON, *THE ELEMENT*, 2009

I CHANGED GEAR IN the old red VW Golf we had inherited from Robin's grandmother as I drove away from our apartment in Wapping Dock for the last time. The sun glittered on the water as the Golf accelerated down the wide, three-lane road that cuts through Liverpool city center. *Wow*, I thought. *This city is more beautiful than people give it credit for.* At the top of the two towers of the Royal Liver Building the famous liver bird statues kept watch over the city and the sea. Legend has it that if these two birds fly away, the city will cease to exist. It felt as if I were flying away through the unusually fine British weather. But Liverpool would hardly cease to exist without me.

Strapped into the child seat behind me was my daughter, who was now almost two years old; I was also expecting our second child. I soon zipped along the motorway, heading north toward Newcastle, where the ferry would be waiting—the ferry to Norway.

"Let's move," I'd said to Robin. I wanted my children to experience growing up in Norway. There was no longer anything to keep me in Liverpool. My relationship with my dad was only getting worse and was now practically nonexistent. He didn't even attend my graduation ceremony when I finished medical school. I'd told him that we were moving a few months before setting off for Newcastle in the red Golf, but I'd hardly seen him since. We never said goodbye.

In the car with me were three suitcases. One of them was stuffed full of books. Another held saris and jewelry that had belonged to my mum, along with photo albums full of memories from my childhood. In the hold of the boat was a container that housed a white sofa that had been in our family since I was nine years old, a couple of double beds that were around twenty years old, and a piano. I've never been very concerned with material things. Most important was my new, growing family—and a document on my laptop. A finished proposal for research that would take me several years to complete.

IN NEWCASTLE WE met my mother-in-law, and together we drove aboard the ferry. From the deck we saw the sea stretching out toward the horizon. The smell of the salty air cleared my head.

"Are you sad to leave?" my mother-in-law asked me. I wasn't sure how to answer. I had the sense of finally being grown up. I was married and had children, but only really felt that I was an adult now that I was leaving Liverpool, the city that had always been my home. On the other side of the North Sea awaited an adventure of my own choosing. *This is freedom*, I thought.

I was completely exhausted by my pregnancy, my final exams, and all the preparations we'd had to make for the move. But now that my mother-in-law was with us I could finally relax in the cabin. As I lay there and dozed, I began to look forward instead of looking back. I still hadn't completed my mandatory residency period as a junior doctor, so I'd do that in Norway. But I also wanted to get started on my PhD straightaway. I'd already checked out the opportunities available to me. As a young, naive student, I thought that it was simply about finding the strongest research environment in Norway and convincing them that my project was an idea they should take a chance on.

Three months before the trip I'd called the head of the department for rheumatological research at Oslo University Hospital. I introduced myself in the poshest British accent I could muster. Would it be possible to undertake a doctoral degree in rheumatoid arthritis and hormones at Oslo University Hospital? Luckily, the renowned professor seemed interested in adding an almost unhealthily enthusiastic doctoral student to his research group. We agreed to meet as soon as I arrived in Norway.

"Don't you care about success?"

THE HEAD RESEARCHER in rheumatology at Oslo University Hospital was an imposing figure. When the professor sat down in his chair, behind one of the tidiest desks I've ever seen, we were at eye level with each other, even though I was standing. This was our first meeting, and I was excited.

"So," he said, looking at me. "Why don't you tell me how you think we can help you?"

I was thoroughly prepared and eagerly babbled away about everything I wanted to do. I pulled a large poster from my bag, on which I had written all the hormones and their connections to the immune system—all the clues I had discovered. "There are so many connections that should be investigated in more detail," I said. The professor leaned back in his chair and listened. After a while I calmed my torrent of words, allowing him to respond.

"So you've moved to the Skien area?" he asked.

"Yes, that's where my husband is from," I said, puzzled about the sudden turn in the topic of conversation.

"And what's the name of the famous author from Skien?" the professor continued. The conversation was becoming more and more peculiar. What did that have to do with anything?

"Henrik Ibsen," I said.

The professor laughed, clearly satisfied with my local knowledge. He continued to ask me about how I'd ended up moving to Norway, whether my family had settled in, and other general pleasantries. I was confused. This wasn't what I was here to talk about. I tried to steer the discussion back to my research.

"Anita, you have to remember that you have a family now," the professor said suddenly, hinting that it was impossible to combine having two small children with a doctoral degree. I was put out. I was sure the professor meant no offense, but to me his concern was misplaced. I was perfectly capable of assessing what I could or couldn't manage for myself.

"I'm sure I'll handle it," I said. We'd gotten off to a rocky start, but I could tell he was interested in helping me. He promised to look into the possibility of me starting a doctorate on hormones and rheumatoid arthritis. I left Oslo University Hospital with even greater expectations than when I'd arrived. Maybe everything would work out just fine?

MONTHS PASSED, AND the process with Oslo University Hospital dragged on. I became impatient. Finally, I made another appointment to meet with the head researcher. I needed an answer as to whether or not I would be admitted there and given an opportunity to complete my project.

The stately professor sat behind his desk, with the light of the clear autumn day streaming into his small office through the window. What I needed was clarification. I'd be able to obtain patients for the study from the local hospital in Skien, but I was in need of guidance.

"Do you think it would be possible for me to work on this project?" I asked.

He looked at me across the desk and smiled carefully. "First, we'd like you to complete a doctorate under one of our existing research programs. You'll be allocated an office and research funds. Once you've completed your doctorate you can undertake research in any field you wish," he said. His voice was that of a boss used to obtaining people's approval—which wasn't so strange. He was, after all, the leader of the most prominent research group in his field in Norway. One with high international status. This was a place that prospective researchers like me would give their right hand to get into.

"No, I can't," I said meekly. The research at Oslo University Hospital was mainly focused on the autoimmune disease lupus. But my mother hadn't suffered from lupus. I wanted to—had to— work with rheumatoid arthritis.

"You'll also be able to investigate the role of hormones in lupus," he said, in a last attempt to meet me halfway.

Saying no would mean saying goodbye to a guaranteed career. I'd already talked to Robin about what I'd do if I ended up in this situation. This was personal for me. If I didn't complete the study I'd been planning for such a long time—no matter the cost—I would never learn the answer to what had happened to my mum. My face must have said it all. I wasn't going to give up my dream.

"So it's all about the science? Don't you care about success?" he blurted.

I didn't answer.

OF COURSE I was aware that researchers often have to make strategic choices in order to make headway in the competition for research positions and funding. But I was also uncomfortable with this aspect of academic life. When I started to dig into all the unanswered questions about rheumatoid arthritis, it was as if I were a child again. There was no bias, no opinions to defend, no research grants I had to win in competition with others. If you're only driven by success and money, you can be forced to put your creativity aside. Then you become afraid of failing, and end up just doing the same as everyone else. It becomes a straitjacket. I had to embrace the freedom I'd loved as a child, when I simply followed my own curiosity. Small children aren't afraid to make fools of themselves. It's only when we get older that we become ashamed of making mistakes.

The head of research at Oslo University Hospital was probably discouraged by my perseverance. With the best intentions, he attempted to talk me out of a solo project he didn't think I'd ever manage to complete. It was a kind of rescue attempt—but luckily he didn't simply dismiss me. It would have been far easier for him to say "good luck" and send me on my way. Instead he showed great magnanimity and promised to provide me with guidance and follow-up. That was my ticket into the professional world of research—a foot in the door. The rest was up to me.

I went outside and crossed the square surrounded by the hospital's pale brick buildings. The electrical grumbling of the streetcars at the stop cut through the whispered hospital conversations of those who were out to get some fresh air. In my high heels I navigated the pitfalls of the uneven flagstones.

I didn't expect to succeed. In all likelihood, I would fail. On my way out of the meeting it hit me that this might be the costliest "no" of my life. I glanced at the pigeons that took flight from the square as a car passed by.

Now my only hope was a small private hospital in Skien, close to our new home. Perhaps they would accept a fledgling researcher with the shamelessness of a curious child?

A second home

I DROPPED OFF my daughter at kindergarten and asked one of the staff if they could tell me the way to Betanien Hospital. I sincerely hoped that the hospital management would give me a chance to complete my research project.

"Just drive straight past the church, then take a left. You'll see a sign for the hospital," said the kindergarten teacher, smiling.

Well, this is certainly different from Liverpool, I thought—I was used to commuting on three-lane roads and confusing one-way systems. The four floors of the hospital's white brick buildings stuck up above the detached houses that characterized the neighborhood. For somebody used to navigating a British city and a hospital with marathon-length corridors, Betanien Hospital really was another world. The brown entrance door was down a flight of stairs, below an unassuming sign that told me I was in the right place. With around 150 employees, the hospital was small, and visiting doctoral students were clearly not daily fare.

First, I met with the head of the rheumatology department to discuss my project. "Come on, let's introduce you to the hospital director," he said suddenly, trotting down the stairs. The director's office was just beside the entrance.

"Welcome," said the hospital director, looking up from the documents on his desk. He straightened his glasses and stood up. "So you're our new researcher," he said, and smiled. His curious eyes gazed down at me.

"Yes, I hope so," I said, self-conscious at all the attention.

"Well, we'll get you set up as best we can, and then you can just get started," he said.

I was given complete freedom, which suited me perfectly. Over the next few years the hospital became my second home.

I threw myself into my work in my new homeland, but time and again I found myself floundering in cultural differences. In Norway, the preferred way to attract a stranger's attention was to unashamedly call, "Hey, you," and though a Norwegian word for "please" exists, I almost never heard it used. As a British woman I was slightly taken aback, and missed the sarcastic humor and refined politeness of the home I had left behind. But I soon set this snobbery aside—once I got used to the direct Norwegian manner, I found it to be very pleasant. When I picked up my daughter from kindergarten the other children would shower me with personal questions in the way that only curious children can. In the United Kingdom, adults would have generally put a stop to these kinds of "impolite" questions, but here in Norway it was a free-for-all. I soon learned to appreciate how the children were permitted to safely explore their curiosity.

As a Brit I was at least good at talking about the weather at length, but in the lunch breaks at work there was quite a bit of chatter about cabins, houses, cars, and boats. I had no experience to share about any of these things, and I hardly understood the concept of having a cabin. Why would anyone want to live for days without access to electricity or running water, using an outdoor toilet? After spending several Norwegian summers in a cabin I gained a greater understanding of the peace that comes with freeing yourself from the trappings of modern life. But early on these cultural differences made me feel that I was never completely included. I even struggled with the dress code—it took several years for me to feel comfortable going to work in casual clothes like jeans and sweaters. There were a number of barriers, I realized, that I would have to work through.

I'd been an outsider all my life, but here the social conventions were different. In England I was ambitious, but this never caused my colleagues to raise an eyebrow. To have ambition was an asset. But when I met other research fellows from Oslo, I noticed that some of them downplayed the significance of what I was working on, speaking of it condescendingly. The attitude of some of my colleagues in the capital was that I'd ended up in a peripheral non-university hospital because I wasn't fit for anything else.

I was young and unknown, with no credibility. So perhaps I should have expected that certain people might shrug or roll their eyes at me—but it affected me. And it didn't help that I also had a long uphill climb before I could even get properly started.

I NEEDED RESEARCH funding, and submitted application after application. I received the odd 10,000 kroner (around US$1,000) from a research fund here, another one there, but it was far from enough to finance my first study. Medical research is hugely expensive, and autoimmune diseases have unfortunately not been at the top of financers' lists. In the United States, over twenty million people live with such illnesses—for comparison, around fifteen million people live with a cancer diagnosis. Still, health authorities have allocated ten times as much funding to cancer research as to research into autoimmune diseases, and the same trend is evident in many other countries.

Managing to grab a piece of the funding pie is difficult even for highly deserving professors. For a new and unknown researcher, it's like turning up in the operating room on your first day as a student and asking to be handed the scalpel.

My dream might be shattered before I'd even managed to get it off the ground. If I couldn't get funding, I wouldn't be able to do anything at all. The rejections trickled in. I even contacted all the pharmaceutical companies that sold hormone-related medicines, but all of them said no. Yet again, I started to have doubts. It was as if someone were trying to tell me something. *You're no good. Just forget it.*

Was my dream simply a great delusion? Who would want to give money to a recent graduate with some crazy ideas few others actually believed in? Maybe I should just give up and concentrate on creating a normal life for myself in my new homeland. If I couldn't find funding, that's what I would have to do.

Researchers generally have to finance themselves, so for the first few months I worked without pay. I had to depend on Robin to support me. The hospital director understood that things were difficult, and one day he invited me into his office.

"How much do you need?" he asked.

I looked at him, not understanding.

"You need to have something to live on," he said, "so we're going to pay you a starting salary."

I didn't know what to say, but I will be eternally grateful for the support I received from Betanien Hospital during that difficult start-up period. Not just because of the money, but because they had enough faith in me to support me. That made it easier to persevere with all the tedious application processes.

—⁓—

ONE COLD NOVEMBER DAY I was attending a course in immunology. Along with some colleagues from the hospital, I was getting some fresh air during the break. As we stood there chatting just outside the hospital entrance, the frosty mist of our breath made us look like smokers without cigarettes. In my pocket, my cell phone started to ring.

"Hi," said Robin, "a letter came for you in the mail today."

I could hear the smile in his voice. The letter was from one of the large institutions that fund research in Norway. A nervous chill ran through my veins. I held my breath.

"They've given you over half a million kroner," said Robin. That was over US$50,000.

I fell to my knees like a soccer player who's just scored a winning goal. Robin babbled away on the end of the line, but I lost track of what he was saying. All I knew was the sensation of pure joy—and relief. The frost crept into my knees. A few yards away I saw the uneasy faces of my colleagues. I got up, red in the cheeks.

"I've been given funding," I said, dusting off my pants. "Funding to start my research project."

Pedants and pests

THE PLAN FOR the study was to collect blood samples from twenty patients with rheumatoid arthritis and an equal number of healthy individuals for comparison. I would measure the levels of various hormones in the blood, as well as the amount of several molecules in the immune system.* I then wanted to see whether any of the hormones seemed to be connected to the harmful immune reaction in rheumatoid arthritis.

---

* We measured twenty-four cytokines and a range of hormones, including cortisol, testosterone, estradiol, prolactin, luteinizing hormone (LH), and follicle-stimulating hormone (FSH). We also measured C-reactive protein (CRP), erythrocyte sedimentation rate (ESR), and certain autoantibodies (rheumatoid factor (RF), anti-cyclic citrullinated peptide (anti-CCP)).

At the time, everything was new to me. I had to find out what kinds of methods I could use, the pitfalls I would need to look out for, ethical considerations and authorizations—in other words, I spent days and nights reading up on research methods. In the world of research, there are bumps along every road. To get your load all the way home, you can't take shortcuts.

I had to draw blood at exactly the right time and in the correct way—only then would it be possible to trust the results. If a patient couldn't come to the hospital, I went to their home. I once made a 125-mile round trip to Kviteseid just to take a blood test at the right time. I couldn't afford to make mistakes. If anyone contacted me to say that they were running an hour late, I would rush out to my car. Just a short time later, I'd be standing on their front doorstep shifting my weight from foot to foot, a test tube and syringe under my arm.

Back in the laboratory I was both a pedant and a pest. The lab staff had to handle the blood tests in a painfully precise way—otherwise they couldn't be stored and tested. The staff at Betanien Hospital weren't used to these kinds of research samples, which had to be handled with different procedures from those for the tests you take at a doctor's office. I therefore wandered nervously around the lab, eyes fixed on the valuable blood samples as if an earthquake were imminent. "The samples have to be centrifuged within the next two minutes," I'd say, gesticulating, when things took too long. If another minute passed, I'd start to look over the laboratory assistant's shoulder. This didn't exactly improve the working atmosphere, but I didn't care. Of all the things that might go wrong, I didn't want dawdling to ruin my results.

But that being said, I wasn't above messing up occasionally, either. The first patient in our study was Linda. She probably wondered what she'd gotten herself into when I took a blood sample from her for the first time. I knew absolutely nothing about the equipment—it was completely different from what I was used to, and I hadn't tried it beforehand. Finally, and somewhat embarrassingly, I had to ask one of the laboratory technicians to do it for me. But Linda was clearly not easily put off, because she continued to take part in the research.

Over the years, I've developed close relationships with several of my patients; it's important to remember who the main characters in your work actually are. Medical research isn't about success or recognition for the researcher—it's the patients who are the point of it all. And they are first and foremost concerned with one thing: how they can get better.

As I conducted the study in 2005, I was asked to give a presentation about hormones and the immune system for the hospital's employees. In a cafeteria-like room, I told the nurses and doctors about what I was hoping to find out. On the last slide of my presentation I had written: "Immune regulating hormones: the future?"

"In a few years' time, might we be able to treat autoimmune diseases by influencing the hormone system?" I asked rhetorically. The hope was that the research I was working on would one day have an impact on our patients' everyday lives. Above all, doctors want more options with which they can treat people—a fact confirmed by the curious faces turned toward me.

"We're probably talking ten to fifteen years in the future," I said to the gathering of white coats and scrubs.

"And so it won't be me doing that part of the research—that will be down to the pharmaceutical industry," I concluded with a smile. While I was fond of dreaming big, at the end of the day I was also a realist. There were limits to what I could achieve on my own.

—∾—

Breakdown

"IT WAS THE best of times, it was the worst of times," as Charles Dickens famously begins *A Tale of Two Cities*, and I could relate to this during those first hectic months of the study. Enthusiasm and loneliness. I was in a new country, learning a new language, working at a new hospital on a kind of research I'd never done before. Despite a certain amount of guidance from Oslo University Hospital, I had to figure out most things for myself. Researching hormones in rheumatoid arthritis was not particularly fashionable, and nobody around me had any professional experience in the field. Occasionally, I had the feeling of standing deep in the mountains calling out in despair, certain that the only thing that would come back to me would be an echo.

Pressure, stress, and the loneliness of being the architect of my own destiny took its toll on me. I'd had my second child, and most parents of small children will understand just how hectic this period can be. My working day consisted of blood tests and restless tiptoeing around the lab; my evenings were filled with books about research methods, major renovation projects at home, and family life. And in the midst of all this, I suddenly received a visitor. Roger Bucknall, my mentor from my student days in Liverpool, came to Porsgrunn with his wife.

I was worn out with worry, whirring around like a hamster on a wheel. As usual, Dr. Bucknall was kindness personified and showed great interest in what I was working on. I wanted to be able to show him that I'd achieved something, but instead I worried that he'd probably expected so much more of the promising student he'd known back in Liverpool. Bucknall was a reminder of the risks I'd taken, all the opportunities I'd missed out on through sheer bullheadedness. At dinner that evening my thoughts churned and I struggled to focus, to keep up with the conversation. Robin kept it going as best he could. *Well, this is embarrassing*, I thought.

"Are you okay, Anita?" Robin asked when we got into bed. He looked genuinely concerned. I smiled and tried to make light of the situation—of course I was okay.

"I just have a lot going on these days, that's all," I said, letting my head sink into the pillow.

That night I couldn't sleep. After a couple of hours I got up and went into the guest room. It was as if something inside me had broken. I sat down on the edge of the bed as if in a trance. In my mind a voice whispered a refrain, over and over again: *What am I doing?* I've never been the kind of person to panic, but I sat there struggling to breathe, my thoughts confused. For the first time, I realized that everything might actually go to hell. And that I had no safety net to catch me if it did.

Judgment day was approaching: the results from my patients' blood tests would soon show whether all my efforts had been in vain. When they arrived, however, it was in the form of a huge surprise that changed everything.

But in order to understand the results, I first had to understand the immune system. How does the army within us function, and why does it sometimes betray us completely?

6

THE BODY
AT WAR

*"The immune system has immense power to protect
us from the ravages of infection through its ability to kill
disease-causing microbes or to eliminate them from the body.
But the power of the immune system is a double-edged
sword. Its power to destroy infectious agents, if it goes
wrong, can have devastating effects on the body."*
WILLIAM E. PAUL, *IMMUNITY*, 2015

T HE IMMUNE SYSTEM consists of a range of cells with different functions, and the birthing rooms for these cells are
found in the bone marrow, inside the bones. Both red and
white blood cells are born here—and this is a maternity ward
that's always busy. Every second, the bone marrow creates more
than two million red blood cells, which transport oxygen around
the body. Each of us is also home to billions of white blood cells,
which must be continually replaced with new ones. These white
blood cells are the cells of the immune system.

The immune system's cells are the body's soldiers, and they
protect us against attack. The classic invaders are bacteria—group A
streptococcal infections are some of the most common to affect

us, causing various illnesses, such as throat infections and impetigo. The bacteria are shaped like strings of pearls and enter the body through bodily fluids or contact with the skin. The immune system would prefer to stop all enemies at the door, but should any force their way in, the system's job is to prevent them from spreading. In order to succeed with their invasion, streptococcal bacteria must therefore overcome a number of sophisticated obstacles and deadly attacks.

The body is like a country, with a military that protects its borders against invasion. The first obstacle that the bacteria must overcome is the fortifications—the physical structures that shield us from the surrounding environment. It's often believed that the skin is the most important barrier here, but skin is just a small part of the body's surfaces—external and internal—that require protection. The largest area is the mucous membranes, which cover the digestive system, respiratory system, and genitals. If we were to lay it out flat, the skin would cover about 20 square feet—the size of a twin mattress—but the internal surfaces of the mucous membranes would cover an area of almost 4,300 square feet in total—nearly the size of a basketball court.

Mucus, saliva, and tears help to wash away unwelcome guests. But streptococci might sneak past these first-line defenses—and on the other side, the border patrol will be waiting.

The home guard

THE BODY'S BORDER patrol has to be able to distinguish between dangerous enemies and the friendly substances that can be let in. Vital nutrients from food and drink are also alien substances—but eating a hamburger or an apple shouldn't trigger all-out war. It's therefore important to have smart guards at the border.

The body's best-known border guard is the macrophage. *Macro* means "large," while *phage* comes from the Greek word for "eat"—in other words, a macrophage is a "big eater." For any *Streptococcus* that has managed to make it past the body's fortifications, the monster macrophage must be a terrifying sight. It stretches out its tentacles and greedily devours the *Streptococcus* as if at an all-you-can-eat buffet. Inside the macrophage, a cocktail of poisons is administered to the bacteria to kill it. There are also several other cells that operate as border patrol guards and assist the macrophages in their work, and an armada of deadly proteins are an important part of these first-line defenses. This is known as the complement system.

If the situation becomes too much for the border defenses to handle alone, the guards call for help by sending emergency signals through the blood, where numerous foot soldiers known as neutrophils are out on patrol. The body produces around one hundred billion of these foot soldiers every day, and they storm to the battlefield the instant they detect an emergency signal. Like the macrophages, they eat the enemy—but with even greater effectiveness. They can even make their own cobweblike substances, which trap and kill the bacteria. But there can be life-threatening consequences if these foot soldiers are allowed to rage around the body over an extended period of time, and so they don't live long. Just a few days after they are born, they die.

There are several types of border patrol guards and foot soldiers, all with different roles. But the purpose of each and every one is the same: to ensure that the body can react quickly, with a broad spectrum of defenses. These rapid-response soldiers make up the innate immune system, much of which is already in place when we are born. This is the body's home guard, which can be rapidly mobilized but doesn't possess the most sophisticated weaponry. All plant and animal life contains this type of defense—it is an ancient system. Similar mechanisms probably existed in the first multicellular organisms to arise.

In the book *How the Immune System Works*, I found a telling example of just how important it is that the body's first-line defenses can respond with lightning speed. A single bacterium is able to divide itself into more and more bacteria, and so the bacteria double in number all the time. It's like the old rice and chessboard story, in which the inventor of chess is offered a reward by his master for his wonderful creation. The inventor says that he would like a grain of rice for the first square on the chessboard, two for the next, then four, eight, sixteen, and so on—doubling the number of grains of rice for each square. A chessboard has sixty-four squares, and so the inventor ends up with a mountain of rice—even larger than Mount Everest. The story illustrates the power of growth based on doubling.

Bacteria multiply in the same way. If a single bacterium enters the body and doubles every half hour, this will result in hundreds of billions of bacteria over the course of a day—the body will be overrun. Without our built-in immune system, none of us would survive for very long.

The armed troops of the home guard put an end to many hostile attacks, and the immune reaction then stops with them. But what if this bacterial troublemaker, *Streptococcus*, fights its way past this first line of defense? Luckily, the body's armed special forces are ready and waiting.

The special forces

EVOLUTION HAS FINE-TUNED our specialist line of defense, known as the adaptive or acquired immune system—the body's special forces. Our body isn't equipped with these forces at birth, but trains them throughout our childhood and youth.

If streptococci manage to fight their way through the border defenses, several immune system cells sound the alarm. These cells rip the face off the nearest *Streptococcus* and rush off to show the special forces, exclaiming "This is what the enemy looks like!" An alien intruder that triggers an immune response is called an antigen, and in this case, the face of the *Streptococcus* is the antigen.

The body's special forces are mainly divided into two groups: T cells and B cells. These soldiers are so specialized that they only attack enemies they have been trained to recognize. A tremendous number of antigens exist in nature—bacteria, viruses, parasites, and other microorganisms—and the body trains special forces for each and every one of these. This is the only way the body can ensure it will be able to defend itself against all possible threats.

Put simply, the body has B cells and T cells for every possible intruder that exists on earth—or Mars, for that matter, should we ever go there. Over the course of a human life, only a tiny percentage of these enemies will ever actually make their way into the body. Most of our special forces therefore never meet their antigen and remain inactive throughout their entire lives, like a Superman flying restlessly around without ever meeting his archenemy, Lex Luthor.

At any given time, the body contains around three hundred billion T cells and three billion B cells, but only a tiny fraction of these are trained to recognize *Streptococcus*. These few special forces are unable to defeat the enemy alone, and so they have a trick up their sleeve. When the alarm reaches the right T cells and B cells, something dramatic happens. The *Streptococcus* killers mass-produce exact copies of themselves, and soon an army of clones is mobilized—each and every one of them capable of sniffing out and exterminating *Streptococcus*. Thousands of clones can be produced in less than a week—and then they go to war.

—⁕—

T CELLS AND B CELLS operate in different ways. When the enemy is a bacterium, such as in a streptococcal infection, attack by the B cells is most central. The B cells produce a weapon known as antibodies, which act like scent hounds sniffing out the target they have been trained to attack. When one of these scent hounds discovers a *Streptococcus*, it clings onto it. It can then call in other cells able to kill the bacterium or hold it prisoner, rendering it harmless.

As for the T cells, there are several types. The first group is the death squad, which attacks infested cells and destroys them. Viruses attack in a different way than bacteria—they have to hijack one of the body's cells in order to make it produce copies of the virus. The death squad can see when a cell has been hijacked by a virus, then eliminate it. These T cells are therefore vital in preventing a virus from spreading.

We also have a group of cells known as T helper cells, which act as captains and give orders to help the other cells of the immune system coordinate their attack. If these helper cells are put out of action, things can quickly take a turn for the worse. One example is AIDS, where the human immunodeficiency virus (HIV) destroys the helper cells. Without treatment, the patient will die because the immune system collapses.

The last group consists of the regulatory T cells, which ensure that the armed forces don't go overboard with their attack. Like a peace corps, they storm in to tell everyone that the danger has passed and it's time to stop fighting. Without the peace corps, wars can get out of control, and so this group of cells plays a central role in preventing autoimmune diseases.

The rare IPEX syndrome illustrates just how badly things can go when the regulatory T cells fail to function. The syndrome only affects boys and is the result of a mutation on a gene that is critical to the normal development of these cells. In individuals with IPEX syndrome, the regulatory T cells fail to act as they should, and the result is a number of autoimmune attacks. Children who do not receive treatment usually die within two years.

The dramatic effects of a defective peace corps indicate just how important it is to prevent autoimmunity. This is also why the body's special forces must graduate from a brutal military academy—and those who fail to graduate are swiftly exterminated.

The training camps

THE SPECIAL FORCES can go berserk and start mistakenly attacking the body—this is the price we pay for developing T cells and B cells that are able to recognize every possible intruder. The enormous variation involved means that some cells might be incorrectly programmed to attack our body, and to prevent this, they require thorough training. The training camps are located in the thymus and the bone marrow, and this is where the T cells and B cells get their names: T for thymus, a small organ situated behind the breastbone, and B for the bone marrow, found within the bones.

The final exam for the special forces takes place at the shooting range. You might have seen the training of special forces depicted on TV—they move from room to room, with cardboard figures representing everyone from terrorists and guerrilla soldiers to old grandmothers and small children popping up as they go along. They have to know in an instant whether or not it's right to shoot. The final exam that our immune cells are put through takes a similar format—only the cardboard cutouts of old grandmothers and small children take the form of the body's own cells and molecules.

Only sharpshooters who hit nothing but the enemy—dangerous bacteria, viruses, and other suspicious intruders—pass the exam.

The cells that put every single shot right between the eyes of the *Streptococcus* cardboard cutouts will become the soldiers who go to war when *Streptococcus* actually invades.

The T cells and B cells that fire on their own cells or molecules fail the exam—and the price of failure is their own destruction. These are, after all, the toughest of training camps, and the body gets rid of the immune cells that might attack the body itself. This is known as negative selection, and it's the most important mechanism in preventing autoimmune reactions.

But despite this strict regime, incompetent soldiers still occasionally manage to sneak out of the training camps undetected. The body therefore has several safety mechanisms in place to prevent autoimmunity, including controls by the regulatory T cells. These control functions exist to ensure that the soldiers tolerate encounters with their country's civilians without attacking them. In medical terminology, this is known as immunological tolerance.

But these control systems can fail, wreaking havoc in the army's lines of communication—and resulting in the soldiers receiving orders they should never have been given.

The messengers

THE T CELLS and B cells are first-rate soldiers, but they need clear orders if they are to do their jobs properly. The immune system therefore has an arsenal of messengers, who pass communications back and forth on the battlefield, right at the center of the fray. These messengers are known as cytokines, or signaling molecules.

Along with hormones, it was these cytokines that I measured in my research—both are couriers that carry messages from one area of the body to another. Just as our world would descend into chaos if we suddenly had no means of communicating with one another, the body is dependent on messengers to survive.

Hormones are produced by the body's glands and often travel long distances to get a message to the right place, such as an organ or a completely different region of the body. But the work of the cytokine messengers is more local. If I'm sitting in the office and have a message for a colleague across the hall, I don't send a letter— I can walk over and deliver the message in person. But if I need to communicate with a research colleague in New York, a walk over to them will hardly be my first choice. Simply put, the cytokines wander between the offices of their workspace, while the hormones are the emails that carry messages farther afield.

When the immune system is battling the enemy, inflammation occurs. It's vital that the cells on the battlefield communicate effectively, and so they produce cytokines to send messages to other cells nearby. In an inflamed area of the body a storm of communication is raging, with various cells carrying orders back and forth and coordinating everything that happens.

An immune cell communicates via receptors on its surface. These receptors act like a keyhole—and just as a postal worker needs keys to the various mailboxes on the postal route, the messengers also have keys. The messengers are only able to deliver messages to the cells to which they have the keys—which ensures that the right message gets delivered to the right addressee.

Cytokines and hormones are the driving forces behind everything that happens in the body—and they are therefore also important when we become ill. Over the past three decades, researchers of autoimmune diseases have turned their attention to cytokines; there are hundreds of different types that initiate various reactions within the body. In my research, one cytokine was particularly important: a cytokine known as tumor necrosis factor, or TNF.

TNF is the most important messenger in rheumatoid arthritis. It holds a senior position among the cytokines and manages important parts of the inflammatory response. In rheumatoid arthritis, the TNF messengers become hooligans that whip the immune system into a frenzy, forcing it to work harder. These rabble-rousers cause inflammation in areas where there is no need for it, and a formerly healthy person will start to experience painfully swollen joints. The TNF messengers goad the cells of the immune system into attacking more and more of the body's joints, and so the rheumatoid arthritis spreads.

But these hooligan messengers are acting on the orders of their superiors—so who exactly is the head of this autoimmune mafia, the Godfather pulling the strings? As yet, we don't know. But finding him could be a critical piece of the puzzle in helping us to identify the cause of rheumatoid arthritis.

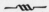

IN SUMMARY, WE have an immune system that we are born with—our home guard—which responds with lightning speed when our body comes under attack. When the home guard is unable to defeat invaders alone, the body also has an arsenal of special forces with more sophisticated weaponry—the T cells and B cells. These are trained throughout our childhood and youth, making the immune system stronger and stronger over the first years of life.[†]

---

† The immune system is one of the body's most complicated networks, and this chapter is therefore by necessity a gross oversimplification. The system contains a range of other cells and molecules with far more functions than I am able to describe here, and the communication between them is extremely complex. Researchers are still striving to understand the intricate interactions that take place within the immune system.

Because the T cells and B cells are so highly specialized, there is always the risk that mistakes might be made. The body may start to attack itself. The immune system has a number of control mechanisms to prevent an autoimmune breakdown, like the checklist a pilot uses prior to takeoff. My mum developed rheumatoid arthritis because of an error in this system. Just as a plane might crash despite checklists and control measures, errors in the immune system can trigger a catastrophe.

7

AN AUTOIMMUNE ATTACK

*"The consensus shows that autoimmune disease
rates are going up and at fairly significant rates.
There is huge speculation, however, as to why."*
PROFESSOR NOEL ROSE,
IN *BIOSUPPLY TRENDS QUARTERLY*, 2014

AM I GOING TO DIE? This is a real question for many patients suffering from autoimmune diseases. The woman in her fifties who sat before me in my office that day was this kind of patient. She was an elegant woman with blonde, shoulder-length hair. I knew the disease ravaging her body would rob her of her beautiful features. It would take everything from her. Including her life.

Remaining hopeful in a hopeless situation is an almost impossible task. As a doctor, it's about finding the balance between hope and brutal reality. Honesty and hope cannot always be reconciled. If a patient asks, I answer honestly. Some want to know everything, while others prefer not to know. And to a certain extent, patients should be allowed to decide for themselves.

The woman showed me the sores she had developed on her hands and feet. They would only get worse. Her toes turned black as the dead tissue spread inward from their tips.

"I'm scared," I remember she said to me one day when the black patches had increased slightly in size yet again. She was having problems opening her mouth as the tissue puckered up more and more. Every mouthful of food was a challenge. Her breathing sounded like an old train and she struggled to sleep. Her movements were in slow motion, and it became necessary for her to use a wheelchair. Depression paralyzed her motivation and lust for life. And all the while, she hoped for a miracle. She had systemic sclerosis. In the end, it was blood poisoning that gave her peace.

Seriously ill patients always live with the uncertainty that complications may arise—and that they may not survive them. It casts a shadow over their lives. Some walk into this shadow with open eyes, while others choose to look away. I remember a woman with the rare sore disease pyoderma gangrenosum, which can arise in connection with autoimmune diseases. Her lower legs looked as if they had been attacked by a monster; they were covered in open wounds through which tendons and bone could be seen. One of the hospital's nurses vomited after tending to the sores, but the patient hardly paid them any attention. They were just an everyday part of life for her, something she would have to live with until she died.

Autoimmune deaths can also occur without warning. Peter had suffered from rheumatoid arthritis for years. He was dependent on a wheelchair, and at the age of forty had to move in with his mother in order to cope. He was a stubborn man, who had little time for all the pills and injections the doctors palmed off on him. But luckily he liked me, and we had some good conversations. I became fond of Peter, as I become fond of most of my patients. One day, I sat at my computer and opened his records in order to enter some notes. Beside his name was the image of a cross and the word *mors*—the Latin word for deceased. He had contracted an infection in his elbow joint and died of blood poisoning.

Every time I open the medical records of a patient I haven't seen for a while, it is with a certain degree of anxiety. Death never ceases to instill fear. For a moment, it covers the skin like a clammy sweater. On the way to work I drive past the house of a patient who died after a protracted illness. I think about how that house, too, will be filled with grief mixed with relief—just as our house was when my mum died. Relief that the suffering is over.

These stories are also stories of the immune system—imperceptible and amazing when it works, but a monster when it fails. The killing machine that keeps us alive can also take our lives from us. Research from the United States and United Kingdom shows that autoimmune diseases are among the top ten causes of death for women under the age of sixty-five. The majority of autoimmune patients live long lives—and many live good ones. But death remains a constant reminder of the brutality of autoimmunity.

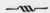

EARLY IN THE era of modern medicine, an autoimmune break-down was thought to be such a bizarre idea that it was regarded as impossible. For a while, it was referred to as *horror autotoxicus*. The majority of medical experts didn't believe the cells of the immune system to be capable of such idiocy after millions of years of evolutionary training. In the early 1900s, the field was charac-terized by the mentality that autoimmune diseases didn't exist.

This changed rapidly in the 1950s and 1960s, when several research teams found evidence of a number of autoimmune dis-eases. The researchers divided these diseases into two groups. The ones that targeted a specific area they called organ-specific dis-eases; an example of this is type 1 diabetes, in which the immune system attacks specific cells of the pancreas. The other group of diseases consists of those that spread through the entire body—these were called systemic autoimmune diseases. Rheumatoid arthritis is an example of a disease from this group.

This discovery changed our understanding of the immune system forever, and cracks began to appear in the idea of the perfect immune army. The body has the incredible ability to create special forces against all conceivable intruders, but some of these soldiers are also able to attack us. Around fifty years after the discovery of autoimmunity, researchers had to come to terms with a new, troubling fact—that an ever-increasing number of people are affected by autoimmune diseases.

An autoimmune epidemic

WHEN I READ up on autoimmunity, studies from the last couple of decades showed a clear trend. Several autoimmune diseases have shown an explosive increase in the number of individuals affected. Type 1 diabetes is the clearest example—the disease often presents during childhood, and the immune system destroys the cells that produce the hormone insulin. Insulin holds the keys to the fuel tanks within the cells. Without the keys, the tank runs empty, and the disease can quickly take the patient's life.

Over a hundred years ago the medical literature was full of descriptions of children experiencing an unexplainable thirst; who quickly lost weight, became confused, slipped into a coma, and died in just days or weeks. This was how the disease always progressed, until in the 1920s doctors discovered that regular doses of insulin kept the patients alive and functioning.

A study published in the journal *Lancet* in 2009 showed that the number of individuals affected by type 1 diabetes was increasing year by year. The researchers were particularly worried about the trend among young children. They estimated that the number of new cases of type 1 diabetes in European children under the age of five would double over the course of the fifteen years leading up to the year 2020. The country with the highest incidence of type 1 diabetes in the world is Finland. In 2005, twice as many Finnish children developed the disease compared with twenty-five years earlier.

The overall picture is not without ambiguity. Fewer people seem to be developing rheumatoid arthritis than previously, without researchers understanding why. But despite the decrease in some autoimmune diseases, the overall trend is that an increasing number of individuals are developing them.

Might this increase be due to the fact that we are better at detecting illnesses than we used to be? Certainly this is part of the reason. Another explanation is that we are now living longer, which increases the chance of people becoming old enough to develop an autoimmune disease. And should you become ill, the available treatments are now so good that you can live longer with the disease. Every year, more people are diagnosed. If those who already have an autoimmune disease are living longer, then the overall total will continue to grow. But although this explains some of the increase, there are other unknown factors that have to be taken into consideration.

Why does the body attack itself? And why are autoimmune diseases affecting more people than ever before? Of course, these questions are related. Autoimmune diseases are triggered by a combination of our genes and environment, and so changes in the environment around us probably play a role. Researchers have a number of different theories as to what it is that triggers an autoimmune reaction.

The evil twin

THE *STREPTOCOCCUS* BACTERIUM is a well-known example of how autoimmunity can arise. Nowadays, doctors often treat throat infections with antibiotics that help the immune system kill the *Streptococcus*. An untreated infection, in which the bacteria are not eliminated, will in certain individuals develop into something worse.

While the cells of the immune system fight the *Streptococcus*, a faulty connection can occur in the system. The B cells create antibodies that are specially designed to sniff out *Streptococcus*. But sometimes, these antibodies can start to attack cells of the heart muscle and joints. Healthy cells are suddenly perceived as something foreign that needs to be destroyed.

The patient quickly notices that something is wrong. After a few weeks the patient has a fever and experiences pain that moves from joint to joint. Some patients also develop an itchy rash; others find that their muscles contract in sudden, involuntary movements. They have rheumatic fever. If the cells of the immune system attack the heart, this can result in fatal damage to the cardiac valves.

Today, improved living standards and antibiotics are the reason we hardly ever hear of this disease in developed countries. But across the world, over 300,000 people die from rheumatic fever and subsequent heart disease each year. The immune system cells that worked so incredibly hard to protect these people from invading bacteria end up killing them.

In the case of rheumatic fever, it looks like the cells of the immune system confuse the cells of the joints and heart with *Streptococcus*. This happens because the markers on these cells are almost identical to the markers that identify the *Streptococcus* bacterium to the immune system. *Streptococcus* becomes the evil twin that commits vandalism and permits the police to haul in its law-abiding twin. Nor is rheumatic fever the only autoimmune disease in which this bacteria is the suspected villain. There are several conditions in which there are clues that *Streptococcus* is involved.

When the immune system is tricked into attacking healthy tissue because of its similarity to something dangerous, this is called a cross-reaction. The cells of the immune system attack two different things because they are highly similar. Researchers suspect several bacteria and viruses of being behind such cross-reactions.

But there are other theories as to why autoimmunity occurs—and some have their origins in the very start of life.

Foreign fetal cells

IN PREGNANT WOMEN, the placenta acts as a transport channel between the fetus and the mother. This is how the child receives nutrients and disposes of waste substances. The placenta is also a barrier against the mother's immune system and therefore protects the child from attack.

In the late 1970s, a group of researchers discovered something strange. They found male cells in the bodies of pregnant women. How was this possible? It turned out that the women were pregnant with sons. The researchers had discovered that it is not only nutrients and waste substances that pass through the protective sieve within the placenta. Some cells sneak out of the child and into the mother's bloodstream. Since the child has genes that differ from those of the mother, these cells are alien substances in the mother's body.

Some of the fetal cells continue to live in the mother for years afterward. Not only do they float around in the blood—they might also settle down in an organ. If they come to a stop in the lungs, for example, they grow into functioning lung tissue. The leak is a two-way street, so that cells from the mother also pass through the placenta to the fetus.

Researchers still know little about the value of this leak; so far, they've identified both positive and negative health effects due to the exchange of such cells. One question is whether these alien substances might trigger autoimmune diseases—as yet, we still don't know. But it is a tempting theory, which might explain why more women than men are affected. However, there are other factors to autoimmunity that are difficult to explain using this theory, such as the connection to infections and hormones, environmental factors such as smoking and medications, and geographical differences in prevalence. So the complete explanation for autoimmune diseases is not to be found here, either. But perhaps there are other things living within us that might explain the mystery?

Over the past couple of decades researchers have come to understand just how vast the number of microorganisms living within us really is. This internal universe, which primarily consists of bacteria, is highly important for our health. Some of the most debated theories about why autoimmune diseases are on the increase are about the impact of this internal bacterial flora on the immune system.

The good bacteria

INHABITANTS OF WESTERN countries have a higher risk of developing autoimmune diseases, and the same is true for allergies and asthma. Allergies and asthma occur when the immune system overreacts to something it should regard as harmless. There are therefore similarities between allergies, asthma, and autoimmunity.

The development of the immune system is particularly intensive during the first years of life. During a vaginal birth, the child goes through a storm of bacteria as she passes through the birth canal. Once out in the world, she will encounter a continual flow of new bacteria.

When a one-year-old stuffs a fistful of dirt into her mouth, this isn't as silly as it might look. The tiny tot is familiarizing her body with an abundance of foreign bacteria and organisms. She's training her immune system to recognize what is dangerous and what isn't. The same thing happens when the farmyard cat drags a mouse across the living room floor, and then goes across to the one-year-old to lick crumbs from her fingers. And again when the one-year-old totters around in the cowshed, touching the dirty floors and the slimy noses of the cows. Without this kind of training, the immune system's soldiers can end up with an excessively strong urge to open fire later in life.

In poorer countries, larger parts of the population live in close contact with domestic animals, and hygiene is poorer. But does this mean that the immune system cells of such individuals receive better training at a young age? Would it have been healthy for me to grow up like my mum's family in India, with monkeys in the backyard, where we would shower from a plastic tank filled with water of dubious quality?

This debate came to the fore in 1989, when the hygiene hypothesis was put forth. The question was whether cleanliness in Western countries had become so effective that we were contracting too few infections as children. In order to learn to distinguish harmful enemies from harmless civilians, our immune systems have to know what the enemy looks like. Does an infection-free childhood increase the risk of faulty connections later in life?

The health benefits associated with good hygiene far outweigh any benefits of growing up in a more bacteria-filled environment, the result of which would only be more harmful infections and a higher childhood mortality rate. The hygiene hypothesis is a bit of a misnomer, because the problem is hardly that we are too clean. The theory has therefore gradually changed to become less about infection and more about our internal bacterial flora.

—⁓—

RESEARCHERS HAVE ESTIMATED that we have several thousand billion cells in our bodies, but the number of bacteria we contain is at least equally vast. Almost all this bacteria lives in the gastrointestinal tract. The discovery that we contain enormous colonies of bacteria has led us to understand that bacteria are not only harmful enemies; the good bacteria we house are vital for life. The interaction between these bacteria and our immune system determines how well our defenses function.

Our internal bacterial flora changes throughout our lives and is affected by what we eat, where we live, the medicines we take, our lifestyles, and a broad range of other environmental factors. Such environmental factors are part of what determines whether an autoimmune disease will be triggered. Researchers therefore speculate on whether the bacteria inside us might be an important factor in autoimmunity.

The composition of the microorganisms in the gastrointestinal tract of a child who grows up in the countryside surrounded by animals will be different from that of a child who grows up in a city. Several studies indicate that growing up with a dog in the house reduces the chance of developing asthma. It seems that the dog's microorganisms might interact with the family in a favorable way.

This research is much debated but is based on a theory known as the "old friends" hypothesis. People have lived in close contact with domestic animals over many thousands of years, but in recent decades we have moved into cities with completely different surroundings, without the same rural proximity to nature. In Western countries, children are spending more of their childhoods indoors. The question is whether our evolution together with domestic animals has made our internal bacterial environments—and therefore also our immune systems—dependent upon them to achieve balance throughout the first years of life. The theory might explain why people in Western countries have a greater chance of developing allergies, asthma, and autoimmune diseases.

Studies show that people in more developed countries have less varied bacterial flora than people in poorer countries. This may be partly due to differences in diet and the extended use of antibiotics in richer parts of the world. Both human and animal studies indicate that different bacterial flora both increase and reduce the risk of autoimmune diseases breaking out, as well as their severity. An imbalance in the bacteria within us might result in an imbalance in the immune system.

Might it be possible to use this knowledge in prevention and treatment in the future? Several studies have looked at the possibility of treating diseases through the use of fecal transplants from healthy individuals. This involves the transfer of the bacterial flora from a healthy person to a person who is ill. It sounds disgusting, but results indicate that it may be effective. In recent years, studies have shown that a quarter of patients with ulcerative colitis experience an improvement in their condition through such treatment. Researchers have also tested it on female mice made susceptible to type 1 diabetes. It protected them from the disease.

There is still a long way to go before researchers fully understand how important our internal bacterial flora is for disease and health. I eventually realized that this is true for all theories within the field—all are currently speculations without clear evidence.

There is probably an interplay between several of the factors that trigger the diseases. In most autoimmune diseases we have no idea why the immune system goes berserk—such as in the case of rheumatoid arthritis.

Terror in the joints

IN THE BODY of a patient with rheumatoid arthritis a long-term war is raging, through which the cells of the immune system finally turn the joints into a bombed-out battlefield. This is what happened to my mum. Cartilage normally provides a protective cushion over the joint surfaces, but it is soon eaten up by the disease. Greedy cells munch their way into the bones. Usually smooth and well-lubricated, the surfaces of the joints become rough.

So what causes this? The cytokines, the immune system's messengers, send erroneous messages to the system's cells, which then start to hack away at the cartilage and bone. This botched communication is one of the most important factors in rheumatoid arthritis. But what causes these messengers to whizz around in this self-destructive way?

The B cells create antibodies—sniffer dogs that sniff out the enemy before clamping their jaws around it. In rheumatoid arthritis, certain antibodies attack the body itself—we call these autoantibodies. Our bodies house all kinds of different autoantibodies, so they also have a positive function. But in my research, I concentrated on those that ended up causing trouble.

The autoantibodies are like a group of terrorists born and raised in our own country. In the case of rheumatoid arthritis, they can be present in the body for years before the patient experiences symptoms. They lie low, waiting for an opportunity to attack. The autoantibodies have to encounter a trigger—an environmental factor that initiates the attack. We don't know exactly what the trigger is—it might be an infection, smoking, or a number of other things—but it is likely that a combination of several triggers brings the terrorists out of hibernation. They first attack the synovial membrane, which lubricates the joint's surfaces and enables the joint to function smoothly. After the attack, the joint becomes red, swollen, and painful—it is inflamed. Soon the terrorizing immune system cells are unstoppable, and they finally destroy the joint completely.

The cells of the immune system can spread the attack, raging around the blood vessels, lungs, liver, and skeleton. The inflammation might also affect the brain, resulting in fatigue and cognitive problems. The entire system is at risk of being attacked, and it is impossible to predict where the immune system cells will strike next.

This is a broad outline of what happens in rheumatoid arthritis. We know a lot about what goes wrong in the immune system, but what we don't know is what initiates the reaction, setting the whole thing off. How important are the autoantibodies? You can suffer from rheumatoid arthritis without us ever finding a single trace of them, and healthy individuals can have the same auto-antibodies in their blood for their entire lives without ever becoming ill. And where is the source of the disease? There is obviously a chain reaction of events that leads to the illness. But the question is, which cell or molecule pulls the critical strings? And not least, what are the triggers that will result in a person with a genetic susceptibility to rheumatoid arthritis becoming ill?

—m—

IN A NUMBER of autoimmune diseases, infections are among the main suspects. The virus that causes mononucleosis (glandular fever, or "kissing disease") is high on the list of suspected triggers for diseases such as multiple sclerosis, lupus, Sjögren's syndrome, and rheumatoid arthritis. The glandular fever virus is called the Epstein-Barr virus (EBV), and most of us are infected with it: 95 percent of the world's population have EBV in their body. Most contract it during childhood and experience few or no symptoms. During young adulthood, the virus may trigger the intense symptoms we recognize as glandular fever.

EBV is a cunning virus that hides inside certain cells of the immune system. For most infected individuals, the virus simply lies there dormant throughout their lives. But the virus may also be able to cause trouble from its hiding place. Several studies show that there is a greater chance of developing multiple sclerosis if you have an immune system that bears a grudge against EBV. If you are among the 5 percent of people who are not infected with EBV, your chance of developing MS is extremely low. In rheumatoid arthritis, however, the connection is weaker.

But there is one strain of bacteria that seems to be connected to rheumatoid arthritis—and it comes from a place that doesn't seem so obvious at first glance.

Over a hundred years ago, doctors believed that infections in the gums were one of the causes of rheumatoid arthritis, and therefore pulled out people's teeth. Rather unsurprisingly, this was not a very popular form of treatment—and nor did it help. The theory that bacteria in the gums were the cause of rheumatoid arthritis died out in the early 1900s—luckily enough for patients.

Surprisingly, however, the theory has been resurrected in recent years. The methods of finding bacteria have increasingly improved, and it turns out that there is a striking connection between rheumatoid arthritis and the bacteria that cause inflammation of the gums and jaw. Such inflammation is known as periodontitis, and patients with rheumatoid arthritis have more of it than their age would indicate. Indeed, the more the patients are affected by periodontitis, the worse their rheumatoid arthritis. It even appears that patients' rheumatoid arthritis is improved if we also treat the inflammation in their mouths.

Interestingly enough, it seems that these bacteria are able to move from the mouth to the joints. Perhaps the bacteria are an alien substance that leads to an excessive immune reaction in the joints? But at the same time, it is also possible that the inflammation in the mouth is a result of the rheumatoid arthritis. Once again, the question is what is cause, and what is effect.

The example of the bacteria in the mouth illustrates that research occasionally provides unexpected answers, and this is exactly why it is so important that some of us think outside the box. I was sure that the significance of the major differences between the sexes in autoimmune diseases was underestimated. The mystery of my mum was still unsolved. But the sex hormones could be the key to better understanding what I had experienced during my childhood.

Just two hormones more

RESEARCH CONSISTS OF a certain amount of intuition, but also a good helping of chance and luck. Perhaps the most famous example of this was in 1928, when Alexander Fleming returned to his laboratory after taking a holiday and saw that a fungus had killed all the bacteria in his dirty petri dishes. He had discovered penicillin— and changed world history forever.

Another example is the American farmer who in 1933 saw that his cows were bleeding to death for reasons he couldn't comprehend. He asked for advice from a biochemist, who found that the plants the cows were eating contained a substance that thinned the blood. The substance was first sold as rat poison but soon proved to have more beneficial uses. Today it is one of the most important blood-thinning medications we have—warfarin.

In other words, it's okay to be lucky—and this applied to me, too. A conversation with the staff at the Oslo University Hospital hormone laboratory, who were measuring the hormones in the blood samples I collected, turned out to give me a crucial helping hand.

The production of sex hormones such as estrogen and testosterone are the result of a chain reaction in the body. At the center of this chain reaction are two important hormones, known as LH and FSH. LH stands for luteinizing hormone, while FSH stands for follicle-stimulating hormone. I'll come back to how the chain reaction works, but for now it's enough to know that I didn't plan to measure LH and FSH in my study. Other hormones, such as estrogen, were what I was most interested in.

But during a telephone conference with the hormone lab the question came up—perhaps we should also measure LH and FSH? It was better to perform a few extra measurements than too few, and so we agreed that this would be a good idea.

To this day, I count myself lucky that we made that decision.

8

JUDGMENT DAY

"Chance favors only the prepared mind."
**LOUIS PASTEUR, IN HIS LECTURE
AT THE UNIVERSITY OF LILLE, 1854**

O NE DAY LATE in the autumn of 2006 I strolled into Betanien Hospital. I walked up the stairs, past the statue of an angel looking up toward the sky. I passed the guard room, greeting my colleagues and the patients walking through the white corridors. For them this was a completely ordinary day. But in my office, the results awaited me.

Most researchers remember the days on which their results come in. Years of hard work finally culminate in figures on a computer screen—and these figures mean everything. Either they're the exciting results you've been dreaming of—or they're nothing. In which case the hypothesis you've brooded over and focused on can end up in the graveyard of science. For me, this was judgment day.

My office was at the end of a corridor on the second floor, just before the operating room. It was tiny, but at least I had a balcony with a view of the residential area on the other side of the street. It was my peaceful oasis, and I loved it. Here I had my stacks of papers, textbooks, and guides to research methods. I had nothing personal in the office—at work, my books and journal articles were my personality.

I took hold of the door handle but hesitated for a moment. My hand was shaking. A researcher is supposed to be unaffected by their emotions—to remain level-headed and analytical at all times. *Bullshit*, I thought. I'd met enough researchers to know that they were just people like everyone else.

I tried to lower my expectations, told myself that the hope was to find some small indication in the measurements—something that would point me in a certain direction. That direction might be estrogen, or perhaps cortisol. Something it would be possible to explore further. I was prepared for disappointment, and tried to remind myself that even insignificant results are of value. To find nothing in particular is also a finding.

But who was I trying to kid? I'd bet everything on a single card, said no to the safety of a guaranteed career in Oslo and embarked on work in a low-status field. I had something to lose.

THE EMAIL HAD ARRIVED. I opened the file containing the results and felt my nervousness subside—and curiosity take over. For a brief moment I saw myself as the thirteen-year-old girl with the encyclopedia on the day of her mother's funeral; as the student asking eager questions of Dr. Bucknall; as the young woman who in the bedroom in Liverpool had smiled and said, "Then I suppose it'll have to be a PhD." This was what I had worked for. Did any of the hormones seem to affect the immune system?

The computer program spewed out figures. Minutes passed; more data emerged, along with several graphs. The connections materialized on the screen before me with increasing clarity.

"Shit, this looks good," I whispered to myself.

It was the hormones LH and FSH that captured my attention—those we had decided to measure at the last minute. When the amount of LH and FSH increased, so did the amount of the cytokines that cause the inflammation in rheumatoid arthritis, including the infamous hooligan TNF—the cytokine responsible for much of the inflammatory reaction. The fact that these hormones stood out was a complete surprise to me—I hadn't even planned to measure them. But what did it mean? I stared down at my desk, my mind going over everything I had read and learned. It took only a moment for the pieces to fall into place.

When the body produces sex hormones, signals are sent from the brain and via LH and FSH. It is these two hormones that give the message to the ovaries and testicles to produce sex hormones such as estrogen and testosterone. We've known for several years that fluctuations in the sex hormones affect rheumatoid arthritis, but all the studies have looked at the end product in the chain reaction—and at estrogen in particular. What if the most important culprits were actually further up the chain?

My patients' stories corresponded exactly with the graphs on the screen before me. They felt better during pregnancy but then got worse after giving birth, and many had initially developed rheumatoid arthritis during menopause or after the birth of a child. The brain hormones LH and FSH reduce during pregnancy, and increase directly after giving birth and during menopause. It made logical sense. Why had nobody looked into this before?

I got up and walked across to the window, letting everything sink in as I looked out at the light rain falling on the neighborhood's large white houses. I hoped that nobody would knock on the door; that no one would call. Pure happiness is best enjoyed alone.

—⚬⚬⚬—

I HAD BET everything on a single idea nobody else was particularly interested in. My aim had been to tread new paths with the hope of helping my patients, but this had involved a significant risk of failure. Up until this day in the office, I had worried I might be making my way down a dead end. For several months, I'd been forced to push such thoughts aside in order to get the work done. Now the worries of the past were suddenly erased. This could be important. Or at the very least, it was something new—the kind of finding I had hardly dared dream of.

Intense inflammation is the main problem in rheumatoid arthritis. If these hormones were an important factor in the cause of this inflammation, it might be possible to develop a completely new kind of treatment for the disease.

I thought of my mum. There and then, all the hardship of my childhood suddenly seemed like it had served a purpose. A warm tear ran down my cheek.

In good company

I WROTE EMAILS to several of the researchers I was in touch with at Oslo University Hospital. What did they think of my findings? To a giddy debut researcher, their response was disappointing. They congratulated me on the results and said they were exciting, but beyond that they had nothing to add. None of them were particularly interested in hormones and autoimmune diseases.

Loneliness struck again—I was on my own. If the results were correct, I would be solely responsible for taking them further.

At lunch a few days later, the department head at Betanien Hospital asked me whether I had "managed to figure out what was going on with these hormones." Despite the response from

Oslo University Hospital, I was still on a kind of high. I didn't want to ruin the moment with long explanations that would burst my bubble of spontaneous joy.

"Hmm, yes, actually, I have," I said, smiling but offering no further explanation.

"Well then, you should submit your results to the conference as a late-breaking abstract," he said, probably well aware that my silence was a sign that I'd discovered something exciting.

The annual meeting of the American College of Rheumatology was just a few weeks away—the world's most prestigious conference for rheumatological research. Thousands of researchers and doctors from across the world would be attending to hear about the latest discoveries. "Late-breaking abstract" is a term used at such conferences to describe findings submitted to the program after the deadline has expired. This late-breaking category is reserved for fresh, exciting discoveries—generally only renowned researchers are given the honor of being admitted as latecomers. I was an unknown amateur, so I responded to my boss's suggestion with laughter.

"Just do it," he said with a sly twinkle in his eye.

So I did, and to my great surprise I made the cut. Of several hundred research abstracts, only around fifteen were admitted as "late-breaking." Even though hardly anyone I had spoken with seemed to view my findings as particularly interesting, there were people on the other side of the Atlantic who regarded them as exciting enough to offer me a place at the last minute. *Finally*, I thought. There was at least one other person in the world who had faith in my work.

I was delighted, but didn't tell anyone the news. As is my habit, I savored my success slowly, enjoying it like a piece of caramel candy. Not even my supervisors knew that I had been admitted to the prestigious conference until some time later.

Throwing out umbrellas to stop the rain

MY STUDY WAS small, and the first of its kind. The results had to be interpreted with care. A basic rule of research is that correlation does not imply causation. In other words: the fact that two things happen at the same time doesn't mean that one of them is the cause of the other.

Let's say a researcher is looking at two Norwegian cities: Bergen (famous for its extreme rainfall) and Oslo. He is investigating two variables: the number of umbrellas per inhabitant in each city and the number of days on which it rains during the year. He finds that the number of umbrellas per inhabitant is highest in Bergen, and that this coincides with far more days of rain in the city. The researcher therefore suggests reducing the number of umbrellas in Bergen, because umbrellas seem to be the cause of bad weather. We can all see how ridiculous this is, but imagine we didn't know very much about what rain and umbrellas are. What if a researcher from a far-off planet where rain and umbrellas don't exist were to look at the results, for example? This is often how things are for us researchers—we investigate things where much is unknown. In such cases, it is easy to draw illogical, incorrect conclusions about cause and effect—and to believe that umbrellas cause rain.

In my case, I saw that the level of two hormones in the blood fluctuated in accordance with the level of cytokines that cause inflammation. Did this mean that an increase in the hormones resulted in more inflammation? I couldn't know that yet. A single study isn't enough to provide an absolute answer. Perhaps the immune system is affecting the hormones—i.e., the causal relationship is in the opposite direction? Or, as often turns out to be the case, the underlying cause might be something entirely different than the factors we had measured.

One example of this can be seen in women given estrogen supplements to ease the symptoms of menopause. Some years ago, large population studies showed that women taking such medicines were less likely to suffer from heart disease. It was therefore logical to believe that the estrogen supplements protected the women from heart disease. But when the researchers investigated this through more detailed studies, it was shown that such supplements actually increased the risk of heart disease. How was this possible?

The concurrence of estrogen supplements and less heart disease might have been a random by-product of something else entirely. The majority of the women taking such medicines came from a population with high socioeconomic status. These women sought medical help more often, such as to deal with the symptoms associated with menopause. More women from this group therefore received the estrogen supplements. Another characteristic of those who come from more well-off social classes is that they tend to exercise more and eat more healthily—and are therefore less likely to suffer from heart disease. It had nothing to do with the estrogen supplements—they suffered less heart disease because they were living healthier lives.

Further research has shown that the connection between estrogen supplements and heart disease is complicated. The risk is dependent on a range of factors, such as age and for how long the individual patient uses the medicine. Regardless, the story shows how what might seem like logical connections are often much more complex than they first appear.

We researchers undertake analyses that can exclude connections being due to pure chance with a certain level of conviction. But it is impossible to safeguard oneself against this entirely. I couldn't be sure that the connection I saw between the two hormones and the cytokines was of any significance in rheumatoid arthritis. But if it was correct that the hormones affected the inflammation, then this was an astounding discovery. And it might help to explain one of the greatest mysteries in the field— why the vast majority of those who suffer from autoimmune diseases are women.

9

THE FEMALE
DISEASES

*"Sex differences in autoimmune diseases
have long been known and are likely in part related
evolutionarily to the fact that the female immune system
must deal with major changes during menstrual cycles,
pregnancy and childbirth—events that are associated
with breaches in the mucosal barriers that are
shielding us from environmental factors."*
ELENI TINIAKOU ET AL.,
IN *CLINICAL IMMUNOLOGY*, 2013

O UR BODIES AREN'T good at maintaining gender equality, and this is particularly true when it comes to auto-immune diseases. Of every hundred patients suffering from an autoimmune disease, around eighty of them will be women. This actually isn't so strange, because there are fairly significant differences in the immune systems of men and women. The female immune system features the same cells and molecules but can respond differently. The reason for this is that women give birth to children. And who are the crucial players in the body? The hormones, of course.

In women, estrogen is queen. This hormone affects cells and tissue throughout the entire body and is extremely important for women's health. It affects the cardiovascular system, ensures that the bones remain strong, and keeps the nervous system healthy.

Estrogen also affects the soldiers of the immune system. Every month, the army goes through continual restructuring in order to adapt to the menstrual cycle. In general, women have a more aggressive immune system than men, which provides them with better protection against infections. During pregnancy, however, the cells of the immune system become less aggressive. This is necessary in order to prevent them from attacking the fetus. The sex hormones are the conductors behind these changes. So when they disappear almost entirely, this must also have an effect.

At a certain age, women are suddenly robbed of estrogen—they enter menopause. Over the course of just a few years, the body transforms into a different one. The muscles and skin become looser, the cardiovascular system becomes weaker; brain function is affected and the bones become brittle. Heart disease is extremely uncommon prior to menopause, and half of all bone loss in women happens during the first five years after entering menopause.

Menopause also affects the immune system, and I constantly meet female patients suffering from bothersome symptoms during this time. In many cases there is no clear diagnosis, but the symptoms arise for a period and then later disappear. These women often suffer with their symptoms for a long time without access to the kind of help they would have if they could be given a specific diagnosis. I believe these symptoms are also due to changes in the immune system during this particular phase in a woman's life. The symptoms are absolutely real, and health care workers should be far more aware of them.

At the same time, it is precisely around menopausal age that many women develop an autoimmune disease. Late menopause will actually protect you against rheumatoid arthritis. A Swedish study shows that women have a greater risk of developing rheumatoid arthritis if they enter menopause before the age of forty-five. The research hints at the fact that a drop in the level of estrogen, such as that seen during menopause and directly after birth, increases the chances of rheumatoid arthritis.

The connection between estrogen and autoimmunity is far from easy to untangle. There are in fact autoimmune diseases where estrogen seems to affect the disease in exactly the opposite way. One of the diseases to most disproportionately affect women is lupus (systemic lupus erythematosus, or SLE). For each man diagnosed with lupus, nine women are affected. The disease causes inflammation of the connective tissue and can attack the entire body. Women suffering from lupus find that their condition worsens during pregnancy, when their estrogen level increases, and fewer women develop lupus post-menopause. That is, it seems that in this case the drop in estrogen protects women against the disease.

For a long time, researchers believed that administering estrogen to patients suffering from rheumatoid arthritis might ease the symptoms. But several studies have shown little or no improvement from increased estrogen. It was also hoped that the contraceptive pill might protect women against rheumatoid arthritis, but here, too, research has provided no clear answers. Estrogen might be significant in the development of autoimmunity, but it isn't the whole answer.

Men also produce estrogen, but to a far lesser extent than women. Nor do men experience the dramatic changes of menopause. But every fifth autoimmune patient is a man, and some autoimmune diseases affect more men than women. So are there some similarities between men and women when it comes to the system that produces the sex hormones? Yes, there are—but to find them we need to look further up in the chain reaction.

We can view the system that produces the sex hormones as being like a factory. The female ovaries and male testicles make up the production halls. Here, factory workers produce the sex hormones and send them out into the body. But a factory needs managers to control the production process. And the most senior manager at the hormone factory is the same for both women and men.

The hormone factory

THE PRODUCTION OF sex hormones is a chain of events that starts in the brain—in the area we call the hypothalamus. Have you ever wondered where the feeling of being hungry or thirsty comes from, or why you feel cold or sweaty? Or why one night you want to pull your partner close to you in bed, but the next would rather blame a headache for your lack of interest? Then you need look no further than this area at the base of the brain.

The hypothalamus constitutes less than 1 percent of the brain but is responsible for a range of functions vital to life. It is the switchboard between the brain and the endocrine system. One example of how much "power" our hypothalamus possesses can be seen in Prader-Willi syndrome. This genetic disorder causes disruptions in the function of the hypothalamus, leading to delayed puberty, underdeveloped genitals, poor growth, drowsiness, difficulties with speech and language, temperature fluctuations, and a range of other problems. The child eventually develops an unusually strong appetite and becomes overweight. In other words, errors in the switchboard have serious consequences.

The hypothalamus houses its own intelligence service, which wiretaps the body to find out whether the right amounts of hormones are present. If the intelligence service hears that the level of sex hormones is too low, the employees in the factory are instructed to work harder. The factory manager's office is situated in the hypothalamus—this boss is the hormone GNRH (gonadotropin-releasing hormone). When GNRH needs to give the order to increase production, it takes the elevator down to the neighboring office.

The neighboring office hangs directly under the hypothalamus like a blueberry—this is the pituitary gland. Here, the GNRH boss marches into the office of the middle managers and calls out, "We need more sex hormones!" We've already taken a look at these middle managers—they are the hormones LH and FSH. The middle managers then dive into the blood, whizzing off to the factory production halls—that is, the ovaries or the testicles. Once there, they give the workers on the factory floor a clear message to get off their butts and turn on the machinery, and sex hormones consequently flow out into the body.

This is one of several such hormonal chain reactions that occurs within the body; all of them are managed from the hypothalamus and pituitary gland. The hormones that manage our stress response are also conducted from here. It was in this system that Philip Hench found the anti-inflammatory hormone cortisol. The hypothalamus also manages the body's metabolism through hormones, which is critical for producing energy. The growth hormones, which ensure that we don't remain in a child's body forever, originate here. And it is also from here that the body controls its fluid balance. On the whole, the hypothalamus and pituitary gland are responsible for keeping the body in balance— they ensure that we stay at the right temperature, produce the right level of energy, remain supplied with sufficient food and fluids, are able to reproduce, and get enough sleep.

What if one of these hormones was also important for maintaining balance within the immune system? If I really wanted to find out whether the sex hormones affected inflammation in rheumatoid arthritis, I would have to conduct a new experiment. I would have to go all the way to the top of the system—to the boss of the headquarters for sex and reproduction.

An idea takes flight

IN NOVEMBER 2006 I traveled to the annual meeting of the American College of Rheumatology in Washington to present my findings as a late-breaking abstract. My boss, who had encouraged me to submit my findings to the conference, accompanied me on the trip. While waiting for our connecting flight at Kastrup in Copenhagen, we sat in one of the airport's many cafés. The sun shone in through the floor-to-ceiling windows as planes roared down the runway outside.

I was completely engrossed in my work, and my boss gently teased me about my nerdy interest in hormones and the immune system. The mood was good, lightened by the relief of having achieved results I could explore further. It hadn't all ended up as just a shot in the dark.

"We have to do a clinical trial!"—the words slipped out of me in my excitement. I'd been thinking about this ever since I first stared at the results on my screen in disbelief. A clinical trial involves testing a treatment on patients—a medication.

"We have to reduce the hormones LH and FSH and see whether this results in a reduction in inflammation," I continued, leaning my elbows on the white tabletop, eager to see what my boss's reaction would be.

"And how will you do that?" he asked. His face took on a serious expression, but there was also a gleam of curiosity in his eyes.

I took a deep breath and took my chance. "We have to give them a GnRH inhibitor," I said.

This was the first time I had put the thoughts that had been whizzing around in my head for several weeks into words. I felt crazy for proposing something so wild. In retrospect, it might not seem like such a mad idea, but at the time it was completely new. GnRH controls everything that happens in the sex hormone factory, and GnRH inhibitors—also known as GnRH antagonists—prevent the hormone from acting. In other words, I wanted to send the factory boss on holiday for a few days. With the boss away, the factory would close. This kind of medication had never before been tested as a treatment for autoimmune diseases. It was akin to saying, "Okay, we have a small study with some interesting results, so let's turn off a central hormone in the brain."

Most researchers would first have completed further studies on hormones and cytokines, looking for confirmation at the cellular level and things like that. It's natural to want to work that way—but also more cautious. My role model was Hench, who had met with his suffering patients day after day and who only wanted to find a cure. The best way to find out whether GnRH was significant was to block the GnRH and see whether the inflammation reduced. Maybe it would make my patients better. I was planting a seed with the hope of seeing it grow.

My boss looked at me, surprisingly calmly, and said only, "Hmm." Tourists swaggered past in the departure hall; business travelers hurried toward their next flight. I looked down at my empty coffee cup.

"Okay," he said finally, a teasing grin spreading across his face. "Who knows, it could end up being anything from a total fiasco to winning you the Nobel Prize."

High above us, a monotone voice addressed a largely uninterested audience from the PA system. Our flight to Washington was now ready for boarding.

The blockbuster industry

THE ANNUAL MEETING of the American College of Rheumatology is like a music festival for research nerds: over twenty thousand participants and hundreds of presentations and discussions over several days. There are auditoriums and stages big enough to be graced by rock stars—it's like the Glastonbury of rheumatology. The program was like shelves containing row after row of jars of my favorite sweets, from which I could pick the ones I liked best. I circled every event on the program I wanted to attend—then snatched my boss's program and marked the same events on his. He just smiled indulgently at me.

I love melting into the special atmosphere at these kinds of conferences—it's almost as if you can hear the sound of minds thinking. But this time I had the added responsibility of presenting my results. I wouldn't be giving a speech but had a large display featuring the results of my study in the exhibition area for late-breaking abstracts. Here, researchers wandered around in the breaks to check out the latest news and talk to those of us behind the studies.

I'd prepared down to the tiniest detail and gone to bed early the evening before. In the morning I put on a carefully selected outfit that exuded professionalism. In the elevator on the way down, a guy commented that I "at least look like a star." Typical for a male-dominated research environment. I was there to discuss my field and my research—they shouldn't give a damn what I looked like. I was twenty-seven years old and felt small and alone among the professors and superstars of academia. But I was there!

When I strolled through the doors at the crack of dawn there was hardly a soul in the enormous hall. I made a few final adjustments to my display and waited for my audience. Several Norwegian researchers stopped by, and many patted me on the back to congratulate me. But they also probably thought it endearing that I was taking the whole thing so seriously.

—᠁—

THE CONFERENCE ALSO gave me my first taste of somewhat unwholesome connections. Wherever thousands of doctors and health service suppliers from across the world are gathered together you'll also find the pharmaceutical companies. They organize dinners at expensive restaurants and throw the best parties. Many doctors can be party poopers, but the people working for the pharmaceutical companies know how to get the atmosphere going. There's a reason for this, of course. Luckily the regulations regarding this kind of intermingling have been tightened up in recent years, but the practice is far from absent.

People from the pharmaceutical companies regularly visit the hospitals in Norway to present the latest research on their medications—with the hope, of course, of convincing the doctors that their medicines are the best. Betanien Hospital was no exception, and representatives from various companies stopped by almost every Tuesday. Unfortunately, they were rarely met with critical questions, and every now and again I had the feeling that they were omitting information that might present the pharmaceuticals they were promoting in an unfavorable light.

The pharmaceutical industry is among the most lucrative in the world, with profits most other industries can only dream of. Every year, *Forbes* magazine lists the world's largest companies, and several pharmaceutical companies are in the top one hundred. According to the list from 2017, pharmaceutical giant Pfizer alone has an annual turnover of almost US$53 billion, and an annual profit of around US$7 billion. They're worth more than Walt Disney.

So it was with a certain fascination that I observed the industry's representatives as they wandered confidently around the
halls of the conference in Washington. They were on the hunt for
the next "blockbuster," as they put it—a medicine that will rake
in billions of dollars, just like the major Hollywood films. I had
no idea that just a few years later, I would experience my own
baptism of fire with the wealthy and secretive pharmaceutical
industry.

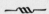

IN RECENT DECADES, millions of patients have been able to live
better and better lives through the discovery of new medicines,
and autoimmune diseases have certainly had their blockbusters.
The search for improved treatments for rheumatoid arthritis and
other diseases comes down to luck, smart thinkers, and a willing-
ness to take chances.

One of my patients whose life has been improved by these
advances is Marit. Her life with rheumatoid arthritis reveals not
only the story of the revolution in treatments that patients have
experienced, but also the story of how much is still lacking.

10

GOLD, MUSTARD GAS, AND THE WORLD'S MOST VALUABLE MEDICINE

"People thought we were crazy."
RAVINDER MAINI, IN THE PRESENTATION
"BENCH TO BEDSIDE," 2011

HOW DO WE treat an immune system that is out of control? The history of the treatment of autoimmune diseases is generally a rather sad affair. So far, nobody has found a cure that makes the immune system act normally again. We have only one possibility: to dampen the flames. To calm the inflammation—just as Philip Hench did with cortisone.

More and improved types of immunosuppressive medicines have become available over the past twenty years, but there are two big problems associated with them. Firstly, significant side effects make the lives of many patients difficult. And secondly, they don't work on everyone. Some individuals benefit greatly from them, while others find that nothing works.

I first met Marit in the corridor of Betanien Hospital. At that time, I was looking for patients for my treatment study, and I asked whether she would be interested in taking part. It was easy to see that she was in the depths of depression and really wasn't doing so well. She didn't want to risk taking part when she might end up in the placebo group—that is, as one of the patients in the study who wouldn't receive the medicine.

When I heard Marit's story, and about all the ups and downs she had been through, it was easy to understand why she was skeptical.

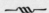

BETWEEN 1984 AND 1989, Marit had had three children. A few months after the birth of her first child, she began to experience pain in her heels and found it hurt to walk. It wasn't anything major—she didn't really give it much thought—but the symptoms were such that Marit decided to ask her doctor what it might be. She was frightened when the doctor said he thought it was the start of rheumatoid arthritis.

"Nobody in my family had ever suffered from rheumatoid arthritis, so the disease was completely alien to me," says Marit today.

Marit's next two children followed closely after, and subsequent to the birth of her third child she also started to feel something in her hands. Aches and pains; stiffness in the joints. The disease appeared with her pregnancies, and the symptoms escalated after her third birth. Marit was quickly referred to the rheumatology department at Betanien Hospital. The doctors wanted to look at changes in her blood tests and X-rays before providing a final diagnosis. Marit therefore had to wait four years before the pain in her hands and feet was finally given a name.

When Marit parked her red Mitsubishi outside Betanien Hospital in 1993, she knew what awaited her. It was D-Day—diagnosis day. In her doctor's office she received the news she had long been waiting to hear. The tests had confirmed that it was rheumatoid arthritis.

"I was happy," says Marit. For years she hadn't been able to put a name to her symptoms. It wasn't easy to explain the tremendous fatigue that came over her when her symptoms were at their worst—people didn't understand. Of course everyone gets tired now and again, they thought. Through all the years in which she didn't have an acceptable explanation, a disease people had heard of, Marit had felt an underlying sense of shame. The freeing words "rheumatoid arthritis" meant that others could finally understand why she was ill.

"It was like a huge weight had been taken off my shoulders. It was true, everything I'd felt—it had a name. It sounds brutal to be happy about getting that kind of diagnosis, but that's what it's like. When you've lived with uncertainty for so long, you're just happy to have it named," says Marit.

In the early 1990s there were few treatment options, and the most severely affected patients ended up in the hospital. Some of them became crippled by deformed joints, in terrible pain and experiencing an overwhelming fatigue that simply refused to let go. What Marit saw in the hospital corridors affected her deeply. She was a music teacher who had trained at the renowned Barratt Due Institute of Music, and she understood that she would soon no longer be able to play piano or guitar. Slowly but surely, the disease would take music away from her. When it finally attacked her larynx, it would rob her of her singing voice, too.

Marit retrained as a special-needs teacher and managed to keep working for a long time. Her family of five enjoyed the outdoors and would go cycling, skiing, or hiking in the mountains—they were the stereotypical Norwegian Vikings. Whenever her illness permitted it, she would be out and about as before.

"But I still never knew when I might get worse. I had to give up taking long hikes from cabin to cabin through the mountains, for example. Rheumatoid arthritis put a stop to many things in my life, but I've never let it get the better of me," she says.

Marit has managed to keep going largely because of the gradual revolution that has taken place in treatment.

A healthy finger

AS FAR BACK as 1990, doctors were fairly sure that Marit was suffering from rheumatoid arthritis, and so the first thing they did was give her an injection of gold. Yes, gold. I myself have seen how patients suffering from rheumatoid arthritis often have less inflammation in the finger on which they wear their wedding ring. Some patients have come into my office with gold rings on every finger, simply because it helps.

In the 1990s, a sixty-two-year-old British woman became the basis for an experiment. She had suffered from rheumatoid arthritis for forty-seven years, and researchers noticed that she had significantly less trouble in the finger on which she wore her wedding ring. They therefore took X-rays of the fingers of thirty patients who wore gold rings, and twenty-five patients who didn't.

Since people only wear their wedding ring on one hand, the researchers investigated whether there was a difference between the ring fingers of patients' left and right hands—and there was. Patients had less joint damage in the finger on which they wore their gold wedding ring compared with the same finger on the other hand. The researchers found no such difference in patients who didn't wear a ring.

To experienced doctors, the finding was no surprise. Gold has been used to treat rheumatoid arthritis for over a hundred years. In the early 1900s, researchers believed that the tuberculosis bacterium was the cause of rheumatoid arthritis. Back then, they thought that gold had an effect on the bacteria. This turned out to be wrong, but the theory was why they tried treating rheumatoid arthritis with gold. And as it turned out, gold hit the bull's-eye.

In 1932, a study of forty-eight patients with rheumatoid arthritis showed that the patients improved after being given gold injections. Over the subsequent decades, several studies supported the theory that gold eased the symptoms of the disease. It was therefore used frequently, as it was one of the few treatments available. However, it took several months before patients noticed any improvement, and there were many side effects. Some patients still find gold offers effective relief, although this treatment is now rarely used. We still don't have a satisfactory answer as to exactly why it works, but it obviously has an anti-inflammatory effect.

Marit's body didn't react well to gold. "It made me sick and I developed a rash all over my body, so I stopped using it immediately," she says. The next attempt was sulfasalazine, yet another treatment that was trialed during the interwar period based on the belief that rheumatoid arthritis was caused by tuberculosis. In the 1980s, several studies showed that the medication does actually work—although again, we aren't sure exactly why. It reduces inflammation and can be useful in treating rheumatoid arthritis and inflammatory diseases of the bowel. But sulfasalazine didn't prove to be a revelation for Marit, either—she didn't really feel any better for taking it.

On the day she was finally given a diagnosis, Marit's doctor discussed some new treatment options with her. Marit remembers one of them particularly well. "When he started to talk about chemotherapy, I thought that was only for cancer patients," she says.

But that isn't chemotherapy's only use. The history of chemotherapy—the very foundations for the treatment of rheumatoid arthritis—starts with the horrors of the First and Second World Wars.

The deadly gas that became a medicine

IN 1860, BRITISH chemist Frederick Guthrie created a concoction in his laboratory that would turn out to be mustard gas. In small doses, the gas caused mild symptoms such as irritated skin and sore eyes, but in large doses, it destroyed the lungs. The poison attacks the DNA within cells—the very machinery of life itself.

Discoveries of potent chemicals have an unfortunate tendency to lead to their use as weapons, and during the First World War mustard gas caused over ninety thousand deaths and injured over a million people. The yellow-brown cloud hung above the battlefields like an omen of the pain it would cause to soldiers. In just a few hours, their skin would become covered in burning red marks that eventually swelled into yellow blisters. But when this discomfort progressed into wheezing and a hacking cough, the soldiers would really become scared. This meant that the gas had attacked the lungs—something that could prove fatal.

Just after the First World War some researchers investigated the aftereffects of the gas on those who had survived. They discovered that the soldiers' bone marrow, where the body produces blood cells, had been almost completely destroyed. The patients required frequent blood transfusions and suffered from repeated infections. This discovery ended up as a footnote in the history of medical research, where it remained for two decades—right until another world war broke out.

The bombing of the Italian city of Bari in December of 1943 is said to be the inciting incident that brought the life-saving medication we now know as chemotherapy into medicine. German planes bombed American ships in the harbor—one of which was loaded with seventy tons of mustard gas. Once released, the toxic load wove its way through the city, and over the following months almost a thousand people died in what became known as the Bari incident.

The survivors became objects of study for American researchers, who rediscovered the surprising effects of the havoc caused by the gas throughout the body. The researchers quickly realized that the survivors' white blood cells were almost completely obliterated. The white blood cells are cells of the immune system, and the mustard gas resulted in the immune system being knocked out of action.

But this time, the researchers' observations got them thinking: Was there something in the hazardous gas compound that might be able to fight the forms of cancer that affect the immune system— namely lymphoma and leukemia? They conducted a number of trials and developed some of the most important cancer medicines currently available—including the chemotherapy agent methotrexate. Cancer went from being a certain death sentence to being regarded as something that could be cured.

During the postwar period, autoimmunity also sprung up as a large field of study. An increasing number of diseases were found to be caused by an overactive immune system. Some bright minds therefore thought that if these cancer medicines knocked out the immune system, they might also help patients with autoimmune diseases. As early as the 1960s and 1970s, certain studies hinted that methotrexate worked as a treatment for rheumatoid arthritis, when used in far lower doses than for the treatment of cancer.

The problem was that doctors were highly skeptical of using a cancer medicine for something they regarded as a benign disease. Patients weren't dying of rheumatoid arthritis in the way that they were dying of cancer. The few scientists working on such treatments therefore encountered significant resistance. One of them even said that he avoided publishing a promising study because he no longer had the strength to confront the continual resistance of his colleagues.

It was therefore only in the 1980s that the breakthrough for patients suffering from rheumatoid arthritis and a range of other autoimmune diseases, such as ankylosing spondylitis, psoriasis, and Crohn's disease, finally came. Low doses of methotrexate kept the immune system partly in check and reduced the inflammation. If the patients stopped taking the medicine, they experienced a relapse with new, ferocious attacks. Continual low doses of methotrexate—that is, a chemotherapy agent—remain the cornerstone of today's treatment of rheumatoid arthritis.

Marit started taking methotrexate in the mid-1990s and has taken it ever since. When she took her first doses, there wasn't much else available to help her. But luckily this changed suddenly thanks to two researchers in the United Kingdom. They discovered what is known as anti-TNF—the most important breakthrough since cortisone and methotrexate.

The revolution

IN LONDON IN the 1980s, around the same time that Marit became ill, Ravinder Maini and Marc Feldmann were steadfastly working toward a revolution in the treatment of a broad range of autoimmune diseases—the discovery of what we now call biologic drugs.

Biologic drugs are produced from living cells or tissue and are different from traditional medicines. They are large molecules,

similar to the body's own proteins. Biologics reduce the symptoms of autoimmune diseases by targeting specific parts of the
chain reaction that results in inflammation.

Ravinder Maini is British with an Indian background and is one
of my most important sources of inspiration. He and the Australian Marc Feldmann made a groundbreaking discovery—but they
didn't just stop there, as many researchers end up doing after
completing a successful project. Instead, they worked with the
pharmaceutical industry to bring to market a medication that has
proved helpful for millions of patients. They took responsibility
for their discovery and finished what they started.

I've seen Maini give presentations. Far too many researchers
try to package their findings in intricate language and minute
detail in order to convince their colleagues of the complexity of
their work. But Maini isn't like that. He talks about his discoveries in a way that ensures everyone can understand. You can find
his famous presentation "Bench to Bedside: Research and Development of Anti-TNF Therapy" on YouTube, in which he gives an
account of his research journey.

He starts his story with a video of one of the first patients who
was given the opportunity to try the new treatment. This was in
1992, and nobody had any idea of the effect that anti-TNF would
have. On a black screen appears the title "Pre-treatment," and
then the image of a gray flight of stairs appears. To the left we
see a woman in a white shirt and black skirt struggling to get up
the steps. She hauls herself up, her hand on the white railing. At
the top, she hobbles across to the other side, clearly in pain, and
readies herself to walk back down. She has to do this sideways,
clinging to the railing with both hands.

Then the screen turns black again, this time with the title "Four
weeks later." It's the same patient, on the same flight of stairs. Or
is it? You start to wonder, because the change is so striking. The
woman dances down the steps like a child bursting out of a school

classroom on her way to playtime. At the bottom of the stairs she comes to a stop, smiling, and throws her arms out wide.

"This twenty-year-old patient was number twelve in a series of twenty patients that were exposed to this otherwise unknown treatment in man before she received it," says Maini in his presentation. From his position at the lectern, in his dark suit and white shirt, he explains his point by simply showing the video.

"I'm showing you this because in medicine there is always the problem of evaluating the efficacy of a drug, but when something like this happens you realize that you really have something very unusual," he says.

—⁓—

RAVINDER MAINI AND Marc Feldmann had been researching rheumatoid arthritis since 1985, when they first met each other at the Kennedy Institute at Imperial College London. The medical world knew that the immune system was the main problem in rheumatoid arthritis, but it was a fresh discovery that led the two researchers down the path they chose to follow—namely the discovery of the first cytokines, the immune system's messengers.

Today we know that there are several hundred cytokines, but in the 1980s they were still largely unknown. However, three important cytokines had been discovered. ‡

"That was a gift to us, because these turned out to be very interesting and important in rheumatoid arthritis," says Maini in the presentation.

Through meticulous laboratory research, Maini and Feldmann discovered that there were abnormally high levels of all three of these cytokines in inflamed joints, and that one of them seemed to

---

‡ Tumor necrosis factor (TNF), and interleukins 1 and 6 (IL-1 and IL-6)

control the others. This was TNF. In laboratory petri dishes, they saw that inhibiting TNF stopped the chain reaction that resulted in inflammation.

But the problem was that this happened in a petri dish. A human body—an entire universe of cells, molecules, and fluids—is something else entirely. Maini and Feldmann therefore undertook trials in mice with induced arthritis. Treating the mice with anti-TNF seemed to protect the mice's joints from being damaged.

"This encouraged us hugely," says Maini. All that remained was to test the substance on humans, but that was where Maini and Feldmann hit a wall. The pharmaceutical companies had no belief in their hypothesis; other researchers thought they were crazy. They couldn't see how a single molecule could be so important in such a complex disease—the entire concept must be wrong.

"They showed us the door. For a year, we struggled," says Maini.

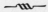

BUT, THROUGH SHEER coincidence, American researchers simultaneously discovered that TNF was important in septic shock. This is a complication in blood poisoning that results in the failure of internal organs—something that is often fatal. Animal trials with anti-TNF looked promising, but the treatment didn't work on humans. The company Centocor had taken a chance on developing these medications to treat septic shock, but now they were almost bankrupt. The head of the company's research department was one of Feldmann's former colleagues, and the company was willing to give anti-TNF a chance in the treatment of rheumatoid arthritis. They had nothing to lose. Maini and Feldmann were given enough medication to complete one trial.

"If something goes wrong, it's your problem. If something goes right, it's our problem," the head of Centocor told the researchers, according to Maini.

This was the background to the trial involving twenty patients that was started by Maini and Feldmann in 1992. The patients quickly noticed a difference. Their swelling reduced, and they experienced less pain and a completely different level of mobility. Their blood tests also showed a dramatic reduction in inflammation.

In these results, Centocor saw a way in which they might save the company and plowed money into furthering the research. Anti-TNF was tested on both rheumatoid arthritis and Crohn's disease, an autoimmune disorder that results in inflammation of the gastrointestinal tract. Larger, more detailed studies confirmed the treatment worked. When the US Food and Drug Administration held an open meeting to discuss whether they should approve the treatment for Crohn's disease, a number of patients attended— this was anything but usual. The patients explained how the medicine had changed their lives and implored the experts not to take it from them. In 1998 and 1999, the authorities approved anti-TNF as a treatment for rheumatoid arthritis and Crohn's disease. A new wonder drug had been discovered.

"The discovery that inhibiting just one molecule could make such a huge difference to the many sufferers of this terrible disease was a truly remarkable find," Maini has said in later interviews. Anti-TNF soon proved effective against an entire range of other autoimmune disorders, such as ankylosing spondylitis, psoriasis, juvenile idiopathic arthritis, and inflammatory bowel disease.

But it was not only patients who benefited greatly from the revolutionary treatment. The pharmaceutical industry developed several anti-TNF medications—Remicade, Enbrel, and Humira are the best known. On the list of the world's top-selling pharmaceuticals for 2016, all three of these medications were in the top five, representing revenues of more than US$32 billion in a single year. This is on a par with the yearly revenue of Nike. Humira was responsible for half of all anti-TNF drug sales, and came at the very top of the list. Never before had a medication sold in such volumes in a single year. Maini and Feldmann's research gave millions of patients a better life. And at the same time, it was the starting shot for the most lucrative pharmaceutical in history.

However, these drugs are not a cure. We are becoming increasingly skilled at using anti-TNF in the treatment of rheumatoid arthritis and other diseases, but it still only works for 60–70 percent of patients—something Maini is careful to point out. Almost 40 percent of patients experience little or no effect, "for reasons we don't understand," says Maini in the presentation.

Hanging up clothes with your teeth

AROUND THE YEAR 2000, Marit was able to test the groundbreaking new luxury medicine at Betanien Hospital in Norway. It cost a small fortune to treat patients using anti-TNF, and there was much back-and-forth about whether or not she would be permitted to try the new drug.

"The question was simply whether I was sick enough," says Marit. When she found out she would be able to try Remicade, Marit was approaching her fiftieth birthday. "I was so happy. It was a revolution when the medicine came out, and I'd heard so much about it that was positive. Not many people in Norway were able to try it at that time," she says.

A few weeks after starting treatment, Marit could feel that something had eased in her body. "Not all of my symptoms were gone, and there was a little inflammation left here and there, but it was very effective for a while," says Marit. But then came the setback. The medicine's effect has a tendency to decrease over time. The cause of this is a kind of cruel joke on the part of the body.

To the immune system, these biopharmaceuticals look like alien intruders. The body's soldiers therefore launch an attack against the medicine itself. Over time, they build up increasingly strong defenses against the life-giving medicine that is injected into the body, and so the effect of the drug fades. That is, the immune system not only causes the autoimmune disease, but is also responsible for ensuring that the medication eventually ceases to function.

For Marit, the Remicade worked for around three to four years before its effectiveness was almost entirely gone. Her doctors then took her off the treatment. She had to manage without medicine for a while before they could try something new. And so the years went by. New medications would make life better for a while, but the symptoms would always come creeping back after a certain length of time on the treatment.

"Every medicine you have to stop taking is a defeat. So you're ecstatic again when something works," says Marit. She's tried the entire range of medicines that are available for the treatment of rheumatoid arthritis. The damage the disease has done to her joints has necessitated over twenty operations, and at times her condition has been so bad that she's had to slide down the stairs of her home on her bottom. At times like this, she needs help to get out of bed and get dressed. For several hours each morning, her body might be completely uncooperative and painful. As if she had suddenly become a hundred years old and in need of constant care overnight.

"I remember having to hang clothes on the washing line with my teeth because I'd lost the use of one of my hands. I always had a bag on my back, so that I wouldn't have to carry things. You find solutions," says Marit.

When her condition became unbearable, Marit would be admitted to the hospital for high doses of cortisone. When Philip Hench tested cortisone for the first time, he administered one hundred milligrams per day—a dose that made his patients dance out of their wheelchairs. This is over ten times the dose we now use in long-term cortisone treatments. But today's short-term high dose is something else altogether. We might administer one thousand milligrams intravenously three times over the course of three days. Marit has received such cortisone boosts several times.

"You have the usual severe pain from your disease in the evening, and you're unable to get up. But then you wake up the day after, get out of bed, and putter around completely fine. It sounds crazy," she says, describing the feeling as pure euphoria. These kinds of high doses are emergency treatments to keep people going for a while. The effect only lasts for a few months, and the side effects can be unpleasant.

"They say it's like sugary sweets—you just want more. After feeling so awful it's nice to go home and be able to function. It's hard to imagine the rollercoaster ride we patients are always on— we never know how effective a medicine is going to be, or how long its effects will last," says Marit.

MARIT'S STORY IS one of many—throughout my career as a doctor I've heard countless similar tales. I knew that there was a desperate need for improved treatment, particularly for patients who are out of options. Those who have tried everything and come to the end of the medicines available on the shelf.

Ravinder Maini says that chance might just be the most important factor for a researcher working to find a new treatment. Fortune had been on my side when at the very last minute we decided to measure the hormones that resulted in interesting findings. But new discoveries are first and foremost about hard work—about running a marathon in which few ever reach the finish line. It's about continuing to run, even when it hurts.

11

GOING AGAINST THE STREAM

*"In school my grades always suffered because
I was continually mucking about with irrelevant side
issues which I often found to be more interesting."*
**BARRY MARSHALL, IN HIS BIOGRAPHY ON
THE NOBEL PRIZE WEBSITE, 2005**

"WHY ISN'T ANYONE else conducting research in this area, Anita?"

I was giving a presentation at a meeting of rheumatology professionals in Skien; in attendance was one of the leading researchers in Norway. Her question was delivered with clear undertones—she didn't believe a young whippersnapper like me could have discovered anything others hadn't thought of before.

"Probably because nobody else is interested," I answered truthfully.

"All the research you're referring to is very old," she continued. It felt like she was trying to make fun of me, but I wasn't interested in arguing.

"Yes," I answered. "That's probably because nobody else has been interested for a very long time." The woman leaned back in her chair, clearly pleased with herself.

To me, the woman's responses were a sign that I was on anything but a wild goose chase. Autoimmune diseases primarily affect women, while the medical world has mainly consisted of men. Researching these diseases has been viewed as low status. In the competitive world of medical research, it's difficult to make a name for yourself by saying that you're researching the connections between menopause, pregnancy, and rheumatoid arthritis. The fact that the world of science is dominated by men is part of the reason for the lack of interest in this area. Hormonal research has the potential to provide groundbreaking new knowledge about autoimmune diseases, but male researchers haven't exactly been lining up to find out more about problems that mostly affect women.

I also encountered this kind of skepticism when I was seeking to publish my results. I thought the scientific journals would welcome my findings with interest, but instead I was met with mistrust. The first journal I contacted sent the study back to me without even considering it for publication. On my next attempt, the journal sent the study out for peer review. One of the reviewers believed that the results couldn't possibly be correct, that I must have done something wrong. It was almost as if I was being accused of cheating. So I wrote a ten-page response, in which I explained my process and findings in detail and illustrated how everything fit together. Still, I received an apologetic email from the editor letting me know that they wouldn't be publishing the study.

Perhaps my results were too far outside the box. Would I never get anywhere without a long, respected career behind me? It took four years before I finally managed to get an article published in a scientific journal. The fact that a young woman barely out of university had hit the bull's-eye on her first attempt must have seemed so improbable that the journals thought it best to pass on publishing her findings.

Stamina

I HAVE LITTLE respect for experts who choose to look down on the world from their ivory towers. They haven't necessarily achieved anything other than choosing the right areas to research—having made many of these choices strategically in order to secure careers as top researchers. But it is history that judges us and the value of our work. I therefore have more respect for the man who won the Nobel Prize in Medicine over seventy years ago, Philip Hench, than I do for many of today's leading researchers at elite universities.

At a conference, I met a Swedish professor who had known Hench. I told him how much I admired Hench and his work, and the professor nodded in recognition. "He was a fantastic man, but when he realized that cortisone wasn't a cure, he became very depressed," the professor said. Of course it was sad to hear this, but there was also something reassuring about it. Instead of celebrating his Nobel Prize and enjoying the rest of his life as a living legend of medical research, Hench was sad that he hadn't done enough. I call that the right kind of motivation—that is, concern for the health of one's patients.

Another person I looked up to was the Australian researcher Barry Marshall. In the 1980s, Marshall and his colleague Robin Warren discovered that a bacterium, *Helicobacter pylori*, causes stomach ulcers. At the time, it was accepted as fact that stomach ulcers were a result of stress—a lifestyle disease—and the pair therefore encountered significant skepticism and resistance. On the Nobel Prize website, Marshall explains why he was so intent on proving he was right: "If I was right, then treatment for ulcer disease would be revolutionized. It would be simple, cheap and it would be a cure. It seemed to me that for the sake of patients this research had to be fast tracked."

Marshall describes how frustrating it was to receive so much negative feedback. Many of his fellow researchers didn't believe him, and he was ridiculed. In order to prove that the bacterium caused peptic ulcers, he would need a guinea pig. He therefore drank a shot of the bacteria to see what would happen. Just a few days later, he developed intense stomach inflammation and was severely ill. "I had a successful infection, I had proved my point," Marshall writes.

Only in the 1990s did the findings finally gain support, and consequently stomach ulcers could be effectively treated using antibiotics. In 2005, the unwavering researchers were awarded the Nobel Prize in Medicine. Putting forth new ideas is a demanding task—especially when they challenge the existing thinking of those who hold the power within one's field. It's fascinating how certain individuals have to regularly withstand having dirt thrown at them, simply because they believe in their work. And *that* is deserving of great respect.

These stories gave me the courage to stand my ground when I encountered resistance. I have absolutely nothing against critical questions, because that's how science should work. But when people in positions of authority look down on others, and seek to dominate and suppress them just because they're new to the field—that's something else entirely.

It isn't that I was going around thinking I had made a huge and important discovery—on the contrary, I was unsure and hesitant. I knew all too well that it was far too early to draw conclusions; that much more research needed to be done. This was precisely why I needed curiosity and encouraging words from the experienced professors I encountered—not just skepticism and condescension.

It has to be possible to test original ideas, despite the fact they often turn out to be wrong. Because every once in a while, they turn out to be right.

A bed of paper

ENTHUSIASM AND THE desire to discover something kept me going. If I was going to undertake a clinical study in which I tested a medicine, I would once again have to do all the work myself. In a way, I was comfortable working alone—it was a relief not to have too many cooks in the research kitchen. But the problem was that I had zero experience in conducting this kind of study.

I would have to start from the ground up. What kind of approvals would I need; what applications would I need to submit; what kind of methods would be the most appropriate? I read and read, systemized and structured. It took days and weeks, and I quickly realized that I would have to put everything other than work and family on hold. I cut out my social life, put a stop to all work on the house that could wait, and worked through the nights. My office floor was a sea of paper. Some nights I even slept on it, like a caricature of an overworked pencil pusher.

Between my reading and note-taking I would sneak out onto the balcony to smoke nightly cigarettes in order to stay awake. I didn't usually smoke, but there was a meditative calm to standing out there in the dark with a smoky red glow to cling to.

The experiment I wanted to perform really was an experiment. I wanted to block an important hormone in the brain. In order to do that, I would have to give my patients a GnRH inhibitor. Much of the communication that occurs within the body happens via receptors. GnRH receptors are located on the surfaces of the body's cells and act like keyholes. GnRH has to have the correct key in order to communicate with the hormones in the pituitary gland, LH and FSH. A GnRH inhibitor is like a key that breaks off while in the keyhole, thereby blocking it. GnRH is then unable to enter the keyhole, and can't get any messages through. This is how the medication stops the entire chain reaction that results in the production of sex hormones.

GnRH inhibitors, or antagonists, are mostly used as a treatment for prostate cancer, in which the sex hormone testosterone acts as food for the prostate cancer cells. A GnRH inhibitor stops the production of testosterone in men, while in women it stops the production of estrogen. These medications are also used to control ovulation in assisted reproductive procedures.

The medication was available, but nobody had ever tested it on rheumatoid arthritis. I was afraid I would be rejected by the ethics committee and the other authorities who would have to consider my application. I was therefore hugely relieved when they quickly gave me the most important approvals I needed—they were willing to let a twenty-seven-year-old newbie test out her odd idea. Just imagine!

But I was also frustrated that everyone around me seemed so laid-back. I thought it might be possible to discover a new treatment for rheumatoid arthritis—a potential breakthrough. Of course we had to check it out, I thought. So why did nobody else seem to feel the same way? It was a real clash of expectations.

Yet again, that old feeling began to creep over me—the fear that I might not succeed. That I was simply kidding myself by thinking this was something important. Someone had to tell me that this was worth pursuing—that indeed, yes, this was truly exciting. All the shrugging shoulders were starting to wear me down.

In a desperate attempt to find someone to talk to—someone who would understand—I googled "GnRH" and started to read. The man who discovered the hormone in 1977 was named Andrew Schally. According to Wikipedia, he was born in 1926. *Hmm*, I thought—*there's no date of death*. He was still alive. Here was at least one person with a true interest in GnRH. I might as well try to give him a call.

12

A NOBEL PRIZE WINNER ANSWERS THE PHONE

"You just simply don't collaborate—it's a race."
ANDREW SCHALLY, QUOTED IN *THE NOBEL DUEL*
BY NICHOLAS WADE, 1981

I SAT THERE WITH the telephone receiver in my hand. Hesitated. I hadn't even dared to introduce myself to my idol Ravinder Maini when I once found myself standing right next to him at a scientific conference. Was I really about to call a Nobel Prize winner? My desk was covered in meticulous notes detailing everything I planned to say if someone answered. It probably wouldn't happen—but just imagine if I were to get a few seconds on the phone with Andrew Schally.

I had read the wild story of the intense, twenty-year-long research race to be the first to make a groundbreaking discovery—and to consequently achieve the status of a living legend. When I read about Schally, the word "dedicated" took on a whole new meaning. His story is the tale of a Polish refugee, an archenemy, one million pig brains—and a tremendous amount of hard work.

Hormones in the brain

IN THE 1940S, the British researcher Geoffrey Harris put forth a radical theory. He believed that the hypothalamus controlled the pituitary gland via hormones; his theory posited that the hypothalamus acted like a hormone-producing gland. But the idea wasn't well received among brain researchers—surely this important part of the brain couldn't be something as ordinary as a gland? In order to prove the theory, it would be necessary to find hormones in the hypothalamus, investigate what they looked like, and prove that they actually acted as hormones.

Two researchers staked their entire careers on Harris's idea— and this was the starting point for a relentless search for hormones that may or may not exist. The race was between Roger Guillemin, a sophisticated Frenchman who had moved to the United States, and Andrew Schally. The heated competition between the two is described in the book *The Nobel Duel* by journalist Nicholas Wade. Whereas Guillemin polished his rhetoric in a way that turned insults and arrogance into an art form, Schally was brutally honest in his interactions with colleagues and others. He rarely minced his words.

When Schally was young, he and his parents were forced to flee the advancing Nazi troops in Poland and eventually ended up in the United States. Early in his research career, Schally worked under Guillemin in Houston. According to Schally, a mutual animosity developed between the pair even then.

"I could not stand him, he could not stand me," says Schally in Wade's book. In 1962, after five years, Schally left the collaboration to become the head of his own research department in New Orleans.

But the pair also shared some traits—they were both industrious and stubborn. The idea that there might be such a close interaction between the central nervous system and hormones was a revolutionary one. Both Schally and Guillemin knew that if it were true, whoever found the hormones first would be ensured a place in the history books.

Geoffrey Harris's theory was that the hypothalamus controlled a number of important functions in the body through a chain reaction of hormones. The disputed hormones in the hypothalamus were named the releasing hormones. According to Harris's theory, the chain reaction was initiated through the release of hormones in the pituitary gland. But finding them was like looking for a needle in a haystack. Of course looking for the hormones in actual human brains was out of the question, so they would have to make do with the next best thing—animal brains. Guillemin chose sheep's brains, while Schally opted for those of pigs.

"Only a meat-eating civilization could solve the problem of the hypothalamic releasing factors," wrote Nicholas Wade in *The Nobel Duel*. Never before had it been so important for researchers to have a good deal with a slaughterhouse, because the hormones they were looking for were well hidden. Only tiny amounts of the hormones are present in the hypothalamus, and the researchers had to be able to extract a certain volume of the substances in order to study their structure and prove that they were indeed hormones.

Schally described that he was only able to extract 2.8 milligrams of one of the hormones from 100,000 pig brains. Over the course of the subsequent laboratory tests, less and less of the valuable substance remained. Once it ran out, there was only one thing to do—get back to the work of extracting more of the substance from tens of thousands of new pig brains. The meat manufacturer Oscar Mayer slaughtered around ten thousand pigs every single day and supplied over a million pig brains to Schally's research alone. Over the course of several years, Guillemin and Schally meticulously dissected the brains of pigs and sheep in their search for the hormone, both researchers doing nothing but work and sleep. There was no time for much else.

In 1969, both researchers succeeded in isolating one of the stubbornly evasive hormones—that which controls the metabolism via the thyroid gland—almost simultaneously. Schally and Guillemin published their findings only six days apart—but Schally was first. After fourteen years of intensive work, he won the race by just a few days. A couple of years later he was first again, when he discovered another hormone in the hypothalamus. This was the hormone that would eventually be named GnRH, and it is the discovery that Schally regards as his greatest triumph—not least because of his victory over his archenemy. He announced his discovery of GnRH at a conference—with Guillemin present in the audience.

"It was one of the most joyous moments in my life," said Schally.

In 1977, Schally and Guillemin shared the Nobel Prize in Medicine for the discovery of the releasing hormones. Their work changed our understanding of the brain—as well as our understanding of just how important hormones really are.

A confined danger?

THE MORE I read about the chief regulating hormone GnRH, the more engrossed I became. GnRH has to be the most fascinating molecule in the body, despite its diminutive size. Much of the human body is made up of proteins—the body's building blocks. A protein is a chain of amino acids. The number and order of the amino acids determines how the protein functions. Large proteins consist of tens of thousands of amino acids; GnRH is composed of just ten. As it has such a small number of amino acids, we don't call it a protein, but a peptide.

Despite its unassuming size, GnRH is what controls reproduction. This tiny peptide is the foundation of our very existence.

GnRH is produced by nerve cells in the hypothalamus. These nerve cells collaborate closely with the limbic system, the brain's emotional center. GnRH is released around the clock in a slow pulse. This means that there isn't a constant flow of the hormone from the hypothalamus to the pituitary gland, but rather spurts of it, delivered at regular intervals.

I noted one thing in particular: the system is situated in its own little bubble. In order to transport GnRH, the body has created an entirely separate set of small blood vessels between the hypothalamus and the pituitary gland. This microcirculation system is sealed off from the rest of the body, almost like a high-security prison for especially dangerous prisoners.

GnRH is an ancient hormone that is found in a number of species, including the lamprey, a kind of jawless fish that looks similar to an eel. Lampreys have existed for over three hundred million years, and have changed little since they first appeared. For a species to survive for so long, its reproduction has to be effective. The lamprey's way of passing on its genes is dramatic: after the fish has laid thousands of eggs, its immune system collapses and it dies. Like a menopause at turbo speed, which ends in death.

Lampreys fascinated me, because in their case, GnRH is not confined within a closed system as it is in humans. The hormone flows freely around the fish's body. This indicates that evolution has taken GnRH in various directions, and for us humans it has ended up enclosed within specially constructed walls. Things in nature rarely happen without a reason, and so this confining of GnRH must be of some benefit. In 1980, Richard M. Sharpe pointed out this phenomenon in an article published in *Nature*.

GnRH has an impact outside the closed system of the brain. But it is obviously important to prevent a continual flow of the hormone seeping out of the brain and into the rest of the body. Why is the body so terrified that the hormone might escape from its enclosure?

There are medications that stimulate increased production of GnRH, and these reveal something interesting. GnRH-stimulating medicines increase your chances of developing an autoimmune disease. In assisted reproduction, doctors stimulate the production of GnRH, and studies show that patients with multiple sclerosis have an increased risk of relapse when undertaking such treatment. Might a GnRH inhibitor have the opposite effect? In a study undertaken on mice with induced lupus, researchers saw that potent GnRH drugs worsened the disease, while GnRH inhibitors protected the mice. The GnRH inhibitors also seemed to protect the mice from developing type 1 diabetes.

Other studies indicate that GnRH affects the risk of osteoporosis and cardiovascular disease. In patients with prostate cancer, it has been observed that those who are given GnRH inhibitors are less likely to develop cardiovascular disease, compared to those given GnRH-stimulating medicines.

There might be new discoveries just waiting to be uncovered here, I thought. GnRH's hidden secrets might just bring me one step closer to solving the mystery of my mum's illness.

AS I DUG ever deeper into the literature about the hormone, I thought of one of the patients I had met as a medical student at the rheumatology department at the hospital in Liverpool. She had come into the office with the slow movements of someone carrying extra weight. The dark-haired woman of around forty slumped into the chair and chatted away with the characteristic Scouse accent of the local population.

"Do you remember whether anything special happened around the time you experienced the first symptoms of rheumatoid arthritis?" I asked, as I usually did.

"Oh yeah, it was after getting those injections!" she answered immediately.

The patient had been given a medication she believed triggered the rheumatoid arthritis she had been struggling with ever since. The medicine is used in women for the treatment of endometriosis—a painful condition in which uterine tissue grows outside the uterus. At the time, I hadn't given what she told me much thought. But I now understood that even back then, she might have given me the answer I'd spent so long searching for.

The medication the woman had been prescribed was a GnRH-stimulating medicine. It may well be that the woman from Liverpool was right in suspecting that the injections she was given had inadvertently triggered her rheumatoid arthritis.

"It's Andrew"

I KNEW ENOUGH to want to keep going, but I needed some support. Surely Andrew Schally would be interested in an experiment to block GnRH in an autoimmune disease—this was, after all, a completely new idea linked to the hormone he had discovered. Usually I would have sent an email to ask whether it was okay to get in touch, but I was impatient.

I clutched the telephone receiver expectantly. What if he thought my idea sounded completely ridiculous? At that moment, he was my only hope of support. I was in desperate need of a positive boost to give me the will to carry on; I had to take the chance.

I punched the number into the phone and let out a sigh, my index finger resting on the last digit. On the other side of the Atlantic, in an office at the University of Miami, the telephone rang. It felt as if my future was on the line. Then someone picked up the phone.

"It's Andrew."

I almost fell out of my chair, completely unprepared that it might be Schally himself who answered. *Get a grip, Anita, this is your chance*, I thought. I pulled out the poshest British accent I could muster.

"Hi, this is Anita Kåss, a scientist from Norway." I had just a few seconds to get his attention. Of course he would hardly care who I was, but I thought that if my idea truly was interesting—something that would set his mind working—then I might get through to this creative thinker.

"Do you think it's possible to reduce inflammation in autoimmune disease by inhibiting GnRH?" I asked.

"Yes," Schally answered immediately. Even over the phone it's sometimes possible to sense someone's mental cogs turning. He told me he had observed something similar in cancer treatments, which he had been researching for years. "It sounds like an exciting opportunity and a good idea," he said.

I didn't say very much, but felt my grin growing wider and wider. He believed in me! I felt like a fourteen-year-old girl who had just attempted to call Justin Bieber to discuss a school project she was doing about him—it was as if he'd actually picked up and agreed to answer a few questions.

"Send me the protocol for the study and I'll take a look," Schally said. The fact that he would take the time to read through the study protocol of a completely unknown researcher from a city he'd never heard of was quite simply unbelievable. Considering everything I had read about Schally's somewhat fiery conduct toward his colleagues and others, I had expected a certain amount of arrogance. Instead, I was met with a true sense of wonder at a scientific problem.

Schally gave me the green light. The study I had planned looked good, he said. It was exactly what I needed to hear. I now had the support of a scientist who understood what I was doing better than anyone else. Now all I had to do was get started.

A fortunate gift

BRIEFLY PUT, I planned to do the following. I would need to find a hundred patients with rheumatoid arthritis to take part in what we call a randomized controlled trial. Half of the patients would be given a medication that inhibited GnRH, while the other half would be given a placebo. If a new medicine is to be regarded as effective, it must have a greater effect than the placebo. Otherwise, you might as well just give patients a sugar pill—the result would be the same.

"Randomized" means that patients are allocated to one of the two groups by chance. The drawing of lots determines whether each participant will receive the medicine or the placebo. We also blind the study. This means that neither the patients nor the researchers know which patients are being given what. This information is only revealed once the study has been completed. If patients know whether they are being given the medicine or the placebo, this will result in a greater placebo response among the group who know that they are being given an actual medicine. Blinding is therefore extremely important. Such randomized controlled trials are the gold standard when researching medical treatments.

Medicines are expensive, so pharmaceutical companies are somewhat reluctant to give them away for free, even to researchers. In most treatment studies, the medication itself is one of the biggest expenses—the cost can be so great that some studies end up being shelved. I needed medicines costing millions of Norwegian kroner—hundreds of thousands of US dollars—and I had no funding. So what was I going to do?

I was still in contact with Schally, and I told him which medicine I wanted to use. The company Aeterna Zentaris sold this medicine, and Schally had contacts there. He promised to have a chat with them.

That same evening my family and I were out at a pizza restaurant in Oslo when my cell phone rang. The man on the end of the line introduced himself as Dr. Jurgen Engel, one of Aeterna Zentaris's top bosses.

"How much do you need?" Engel asked. He was clearly a busy man of few words. It sounded as if this was just another item on his to-do list that he was fitting in between other things. Bewildered, I explained how many doses I would need to complete the study.

"Okay, Anita. We'll send it over to you. Bye for now!" I sat there with my plate of half-eaten pizza, staring at my phone. It was as if someone had spoken to me from Mars. I'd just been given medications worth millions of kroner by a person I'd never even met. He had asked me no other questions. Schally must've really had faith in my project, as he had clearly convinced Engel to send this incredibly expensive medicine to a small, unknown city in Norway.

With the medication in place I had removed one of my biggest hurdles. Now I needed to find a hundred patients, which would be no easy task. I would start treating the first patient in the autumn of 2008, and it would take several years to complete the study. At the same time, dramatic changes were taking place at home.

A sole parent

IT WAS THURSDAY, October 2, 2008. Robin came home and said he had news. He was head of the local branch of the Labour Party and had attracted attention higher up in the party ranks. The Labour Party were currently in power, and they had Robin earmarked for the position of state secretary in the Ministry of Petroleum and Energy. The job would involve working long days and Robin's constant presence in Oslo, a two-hour drive from our home in Porsgrunn.

"Starting next Monday I'll only be home on weekends," said Robin.

We had two children, and I thought about how I would cope as their sole parent during the week, with a huge research project currently in its infancy and a residency still to complete. In a country that still felt foreign to me. When I finally got a quiet moment to myself, I started to cry. I don't cry very often, and so I clearly remember the few occasions on which I have.

My life had been full of upheaval since childhood. You learn to adapt, to make things work, despite the difficult circumstances. Strict prioritization and structure were the solution. Between work, commuting, cooking, playtime, and caring for the children, I learned to clear snow with a child on my back and how to make a playhouse in the garden. I used the nights to keep on top of things at work.

Robin traveled often with work. Once, he'd been abroad for a couple of weeks when he hurried in the front door with his phone to his ear. I scowled at him from the living room. After two weeks away it just didn't seem acceptable for him to be more concerned with blathering away on the phone than greeting his family. He set down his suitcase and gave me a perfunctory wave, then walked down the stairs, went into his office, and closed the door behind him. *How disrespectful!*, I thought, tramping after him.

"Who on earth are you talking to, anyway?" I shouted as I made my way down the stairs. "The bloody prime minister?!"

The door to the office slowly opened a crack. Robin peeked out.

"Yes," he whispered, and closed the door.

I went back up the stairs, heat rising in my cheeks.

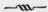

BY THE AUTUMN of 2009 I still only had half the number of patients I needed for the study. It was slow going. At the same time, I started my mandatory residency as a junior doctor at a different hospital, and became pregnant again. With my belly growing week by week I conducted a large research study and worked full-time as a medical intern in the accident and emergency department at Telemark Hospital.

And so the days passed—life was hectic, and we soon became a family of five. I worked right up until the day my daughter was born, and five days later I was back in the office. There, I set up a baby-changing station and breastfed her during my breaks. My newborn daughter happily gurgled away, strapped to my chest as I worked. This isn't something I'm particularly proud of, but it was a necessity. The study was already delayed. I was longing to make progress, find answers.

The idea that I might not be able to do it all never occurred to me. The residency was for a limited period, and the study would be finished at some point. And anyway, the research gave me a kick—I was in my own little bubble. It was a kind of calling that was always with me, regardless of whatever else was going on. On many days I would put the kids to bed in the evening and then go straight back to the office, where I would work through the night before going home to wake the children for breakfast. Robin started to worry about my health.

"People die from not getting enough sleep," he said one day. His nagging irritated me. After all, I wasn't the only one in the family spending long days on the job, and I was doing what was necessary to make things work. That same day I went back to the office and worked through the night again. When I woke my daughter in the morning, she looked at me with sad eyes.

"Have you been working all night?" she asked. I tried to smile and dispel her concern as I took out her clothes for the day. "Can you die of it?" she asked suddenly. She had clearly overheard my conversation with Robin the day before, and now she was scared. This made my heart hurt.

"No, it's not dangerous," I said, pulling her onto my lap. "Mummy's working a lot right now because she has to finish something important, but it isn't dangerous." I sat there with her, stroking her hair.

13

DIGGING DEEP IN THE TRASH

"Never give in, never give in, never, never, never—
in nothing great or small, large or petty—never give in
except to convictions of honour and good sense."
WINSTON CHURCHILL, IN HIS SPEECH
TO THE HARROW SCHOOL, 1941

WITH A GROAN I heaved two huge bags of garbage out of the dumpster behind the hospital, silently cursing the below-freezing temperature that made my fingers into icicles. *What a wonderful February day*, I thought to myself as I stacked the bags on top of each other. When I climbed on top of them, I managed to reach over the side of the container and began to dig into the splendors beneath its lid. The only heat came from my breath on the cold air as I panted my way through bag upon bag of trash.

The medicine for the study had arrived earlier that day—a parcel worth millions of kroner. The hospital staff weren't used to receiving research deliveries and so were unaware of how important it was to retain detailed information about everything— including the fact that the medicines had been appropriately transported. Such deliveries therefore contain a device that records the temperatures to which the substance is subjected along the way and creates a log. If the medicine is exposed to temperatures that are too high or too low, it might be ruined. When I was told the medicine had arrived at the hospital, the temperature logger was the first thing I looked for.

"Where's the temperature logger?" I asked. I got only confused looks in response.

"There wasn't a temperature logger included," someone said. But I refused to believe that the pharmaceutical company would have sent such valuable cargo through the mail without including one.

"Where's the packaging?" I asked.

They pointed out toward the hospital's rear yard, at the huge waste container.

Hospital refuse is not for the fainthearted—it contains quite a lot of bodily waste. This was not the researcher's life I had imagined for myself. At that moment, I keenly felt the disappointment of not being part of a large research environment with good procedures and experienced staff, where I would never have had to dig around in the trash like a magpie searching for food. I could feel my colleagues' gazes boring into my back as they watched me from the window.

Finally, after searching through three bags of garbage to no avail, I found it. I felt like the gold diggers in the Donald Duck comic strips who suddenly strike gold. I let out a silent cheer. Yet another crisis averted.

Tangible proof

FINALLY, I MANAGED to enroll all the one hundred patients I needed in the study. I gave them the GnRH inhibitor for just five days. The patients received their first dose on Monday, and the last on Friday. I took their blood samples almost daily in order to monitor changes in their levels of hormones and cytokines.

GnRH inhibitors have been thoroughly tested and are regarded as safe to use—they have few side effects. But putting a stop to the entire sex hormone system has consequences: the patients would be temporarily infertile. Nor had the effects of long-term use been studied in detail. So I was careful. Over the course of my study, I would only give my patients the medication for five days.

Would my patients notice any improvement? I was unsure whether five days would be enough to see any difference. It would probably be too short a period of time for the medicine to have any great effect. In a treatment study, improving the condition of the patients is the main objective, and it would therefore also be the most important factor that we would measure in the study. But for me, another question was even more important. Would blocking GnRH affect the immune system?

When Philip Hench discovered the magical effect of cortisol, he simultaneously discovered how much the hormone affected the immune system and reduced inflammation. I wondered whether blocking GnRH would have a similar effect. If so, it might be possible to find a new treatment for rheumatoid arthritis.

But getting the patients safely through the study was of course most important of all. There is always a risk in giving patients a new medication. Even if serious side effects are rare, they are each and every doctor's greatest fear. This was a safe medication, but it was impossible to completely rule out the possibility that something undesirable might happen.

One of my patients was Eva, a tall, attractive woman who had suffered from rheumatoid arthritis for years. She had developed the disease in her thirties, right after giving birth. I remember the tight, shining skin of her hands, which rendered even simple tasks difficult. Her life consisted of pain, stiffness, fatigue, and continual surgeries. But Eva defied her symptoms, knitting mittens and baking cakes for several of the hospital's employees. I wished with all my heart that Eva would experience even the tiniest inkling of an improvement.

After five days of treatment, Eva came into the laboratory one Friday evening to have the last of her blood tests taken. I immediately noticed that a new glow had flared up in her eyes. "Anita, I've been to the shopping center today," she said, her voice filled with pride. That she had managed to get out and about to go shopping was certainly unusual. She held out her hands with the biggest smile in world. "Feel them!" she said, shoving her hands in mine. Before the treatment, her skin had been like a balloon about to burst, but I could now see wrinkles on the backs of her hands. It was as if her skin had relaxed for the first time in years. *Cool*, I thought. A change I could touch; could feel.

I found it hard to believe that this kind of improvement could be down to a placebo effect or pure chance, but I couldn't know for sure. Only a few patients experienced such a striking recovery, but those who did were obviously better. I slowly began to believe that there might be something to this treatment. But at the same time, I had no idea which of my patients were receiving the GnRH inhibitor. I could do nothing but wait until all the patients had completed the study. Only then would I know whether the treatment seemed to work.

The second judgment day

IN SEPTEMBER 2011 I received an email from the head nurse working on the study. The text was short and to the point: "These are the results from the Norwegian jury." I laughed at the

Eurovision Song Contest reference, but butterflies were fluttering around inside me. The email contained the code that would reveal which patients had received the medicine, and which had been given a placebo. The results—after three years of exhausting hard work. Win or lose. Over the course of several hours I downloaded, analyzed, and assessed the data.

The main objective had been to find out whether the condition of the patients who had received the medicine had improved after five days of treatment, compared to those who had been given a placebo. When treating rheumatoid arthritis, it can often take a long time to see any effect from a medicine. It was risky to run the trial for such a short period of time, but we had to be careful. However, I still hoped that five days would be enough to see an improvement in the inflammation tests. If so, it would justify a new study in which we could treat the patients over a longer period. This was the first step in seeing whether or not the medicine was worth pursuing.

In terms of the main objective of the study— to see whether the patients who had received the medicine were healthier than the ones who hadn't—we saw no difference between the two groups. I was prepared for this. But we had taken a number of other measurements that did show a clear difference in favor of the patients who had received the medicine. Using a different method than the one we used to measure the main objective of the study, we found that twice as many patients had experienced an improvement in their condition after being given the GnRH inhibitor. We also saw that six of the forty-eight patients who received the medicine experienced what we call remission. They no longer had any symptoms, and their blood tests showed that the disease was not active. They now functioned almost as if they were completely healthy. None of the patients who were given a placebo experienced such a remission.

And then to the question I wanted to answer most of all: Did blocking the hormone cascade at the top of the system result in less inflammation? If so, the result would pave the way for an entirely new field of research.

When I saw the results, I smiled. Before me was the answer I had dreamed of. In patients who had received the GnRH inhibitor, we saw fewer cytokines that cause inflammation. And not least, this also applied to TNF—the conductor behind the inflammation in rheumatoid arthritis. TNF had all but disappeared in the patients who experienced remission.

Was it really possible that I had found a medication that worked—and worked better than the alternatives currently available? A dream medicine is something that works fast and effectively, without troubling side effects. Something as yet unavailable in the treatment of autoimmune diseases such as rheumatoid arthritis.

My thoughts immediately turned to the next step. Of course I would have to conduct a larger study, and we'd need to treat the patients for longer than just five days. I was happy to see such positive results, but I also felt the weight of the responsibility I now had to keep going. And I'd now need to ensure that my findings were noticed by someone willing to bet millions of kroner on a larger study.

Pockets deep enough for this exist in only one place—at the major pharmaceutical companies.

It's our medicine you've been researching

IN AN ENORMOUS hall that reminded me of an aircraft hangar, thousands of scientists swaggered around an almost endless range of displays featuring research results. They squinted at graphs and tables, pensively scratched their chins, and discussed findings with their colleagues. A carpet had been rolled out like a dark-red runner across the gray concrete floor. The researchers gathered in small, buzzing groups, as if at a gigantic cocktail party.

It was the annual conference of the American College of Rheumatology in San Diego in 2013. Once again, I had been given the opportunity to present my results in the prestigious "late-breaking abstracts" category. Many of the researchers around me were superstars in their fields, and I felt like the odd one out. Right behind me stood one of the world's leading researchers, an intimidating guy with piercing eyes. I felt nervous just standing near him.

I noticed a man hovering around my display, as if he were trying to read what it said without getting too close. Then he suddenly raised his eyebrows and took a step closer. He studied the materials with interest through his rectangular glasses before waving to a colleague. "Look at this, this is our medication!"

They conversed in low voices before glancing across at me. "Hi, we're with Merck Serono," the man said, taking my hand and smiling broadly. "It's our medicine you've been researching."

Merck Serono had recently bought the rights to the medicine from the company that had provided it for my study. I straightened up, trying to keep my expression neutral. This man was the company's head researcher. After we'd exchanged a few pleasantries he invited me to dinner that evening.

"We'd like to hear more about your results," he said.

The dinner was at a fancy restaurant beside the conference center; around the table sat six representatives from Merck Serono. They bombarded me with questions—of course they were fishing for information. I had to be careful. The trick was to reveal enough to keep them interested, but not to give them enough detail that they'd be able to steal my ideas and start up on their own. The head researcher was familiar with Andrew Schally but wasn't as impressed by the Nobel Prize winner as I was.

"To think that Schally wanted to use it as a contraceptive!" he said, bursting into laughter. Plenty of people had probably done exactly the same thing behind my own back when I'd suggested using the medication to treat rheumatoid arthritis, so I simply smiled politely and played along.

I had stumbled into a new area I knew too little about. How was I going to respond to any proposal the pharmaceutical company might make? I was at least determined not to be charmed by luxurious dinners and informal discussions around a restaurant table. I would need more of a commitment than that. This was an opportunity to discover a new treatment for autoimmune diseases, and such chances don't come along very often. A large study would cost over 20 million kroner, or US$2 million—which I, of course, didn't have.

I would need the help of someone who understood the business side of medical research. And somewhat unexpectedly, this help would come following a TV broadcast.

"I saw you on TV"

TOWARD THE END of 2013, the Norwegian TV broadcaster NRK aired a news segment entitled "A new medicine for rheumatoid arthritis," in which they interviewed one of the patients from my study who had experienced an improvement. She explained how she hoped the medicine would soon be made generally available. "It could completely change lives—mine and many others'," she said. I thought the segment would only be aired locally, but NRK broadcast it nationally as part of the evening news.

The next day I received an email: "I saw you on the nine o'clock news last night. It was a great segment—congratulations!"

The email was from one of the managers of the company Inven2, the largest company in Norway to work with the commercialization of research, jointly owned by the University of Oslo and Oslo University Hospital. I had previously contacted them to ask for advice, but they'd been clear that they were unable to help. As a joke, they'd told me that I "shouldn't buy myself a Porsche just yet." Now *they* were suddenly calling *me*. Appearing on TV clearly helps you get ahead.

Inven2 put two new people on the case—Anders and Jørund. Finally, I had some support in the work to get the pharmaceutical industry on board. I imagined it would probably take a year of work with a larger study to find out whether GnRH inhibitors were effective. But then we made an all-important decision regarding what the next step should be.

It started with a simple question in an email from Anders. Would it be possible to test a GnRH inhibitor over a longer period of time on a small group of patients? That might give us a hint as to whether treatment over a longer period would have a better effect than over the five days of the study. The management at Betanien Hospital would support an experimental trial as long as the selected patients had no other options for treatment. The pharmaceutical committee at the hospital also gave me their approval.

We were ready for our first test patient.

14

THE EXPERIMENT

*"Some autoimmune diseases are life-threatening.
Virtually all are debilitating, and require lifelong
medical care. Although treatments exist for many
autoimmune diseases, we do not yet have
definitive cures for any of them."*

FROM "PROGRESS IN AUTOIMMUNE DISEASES
RESEARCH," A REPORT TO CONGRESS BY THE
NATIONAL INSTITUTES OF HEALTH, 2005

THIS WILL MAKE HER HAPPY, I thought. In my office was one of my patients from the first study—Sandra. She had seen an improvement in her condition after just five days of treatment. She had since asked me on several occasions if she could try the medicine again. Her hopeful face was glowing—she clearly knew what this was about.

"We've decided to test the medication over a longer period of time on a select number of patients," I said. A smile burst across Sandra's face, and I could understand why. She was severely affected by rheumatoid arthritis and had tried every single medicine available, but nothing worked. Her doctors had run out of options—this was her last chance. It would be relatively safe to start with her, I thought. I thoroughly explained all the risks involved and told her that the treatment was experimental. No promises.

"How does that sound?" I asked.

"I've prayed to God that I'd get this medicine again," she said. "Of course I want to try it."

WE ADMINISTERED THE first dose in March 2014; Sandra was given the code name "Patient 1." This time we chose a different type of GnRH inhibitor—it acted in the same way, but lasted longer after each dose. The medication is usually used in high doses in men with prostate cancer. I was careful with the dosage and examined Sandra thoroughly before starting the treatment to ensure that her body was otherwise healthy.

A few days later we did some blood tests. The questions remained the same: would the immune system react to the blocking of GnRH? Did the blood tests show less inflammation? We measured the inflammation by measuring something called C-reactive protein, or CRP for short. The more inflammation, the higher the figure. Before we gave Sandra her first infusion of medicine, we measured her CRP level at fifty-five. This is high. The norm for someone not suffering from inflammation is below five. I've had my own CRP level measured once in my life, when I was suffering from a severe case of the flu and unable to work. My CRP level at that time was twenty-five. Which says something about just how much inflammation these patients have in their bodies.

"This can't be right," I said under my breath when I received the results. Sandra's CRP level had been above fifty. It was now down in the twenties—after just a few days. I checked again. Yes, the figure was correct. It was odd that a number on a screen was one of the few things that could make me cry, but it was an outlet for the pressure I felt in such critical moments. Such a huge reduction in just a few days surely couldn't be down to chance?

"The pain is almost gone," said Sandra when she came in for a checkup. She told me that the stiffness she experienced every morning, which is so typical of rheumatoid arthritis, had eased significantly. Gone were the hours in the mornings in which she would have to slowly knead her joints into action. I saw how the swelling disappeared from her joints before my very eyes. Soon she was able to work more, and her energy returned like a frozen waterfall melting in spring.

In April, I sent an email to Anders at Inven2. "Great news!" I started. "The first patient who took GnRH antagonist three weeks ago has responded strikingly." That same day, Sandra's CRP level was measured at eighteen. The lowest it had been in three years.

After she had been on the medicine for a while, Sandra sent me the results of the blood tests taken by her GP. On the outside of the folder was a yellow Post-it, on which she had scribbled a note telling me the tests looked good. "It works!" she concluded.

The results from the first test patient exceeded all expectations— I could hardly believe what I was seeing. I had to be sure that chance wasn't playing a trick on me. It might simply be that this patient had suddenly entered a period of improvement that had nothing to do with the medicine. Would it work just as effectively on others?

From bed to bicycle

AT ONE OF the morning meetings at Betanien Hospital I listened with interest as the doctors discussed a patient they were

152

struggling to treat. She was a common presence in the department—a woman who had been given all available treatments but who sadly never experienced any stable improvement. She had now been admitted to the hospital for intravenous high-dosage treatment using cortisone—something we do when a patient is suffering so much that they need a boost to return them to life. She was a classic treatment-resistant rheumatoid arthritis patient, for whom the effects of a range of medicines would only last for a short while before her condition worsened again.

"Can we try a GnRH inhibitor on her?" I asked. One of the doctors gave me an odd look.

"If you're aiming to prove that the medicine works, I'm not sure it's such a good idea to test it on her—for this patient, nothing seems to be effective," he said.

"If GnRH inhibitors are going to be worth pursuing, they have to offer something new—and maybe even work for patients who have run out of options," I argued. These patients really needed new alternatives. I was willing to take the chance.

"Well, feel free—and good luck," they said to me.

That's how I came to meet Marit again.

The hospital was full, so she lay in the corridor, in a state even worse than the last time we met. Back then, she had turned down my offer to take part in the first study. I explained that we were now testing the medicine over a longer period of time on a handful of patients. This time, there was no possibility that she would be given a placebo. "Would you like to try it?" I asked. Marit immediately answered in the affirmative.

"There was absolutely no doubt in my mind that I wanted to try it. I was tired of being ill," says Marit today.

Marit started taking the medicine in May. She was "Patient 2."

—◊◊◊—

MARIT WAS IN a very bad state when she was given her first dose. She was unable to get out of bed before midday, was no longer able to drive a car, and was often in intense pain. I was careful not to promise her anything and told her that we had only tested long-term treatment on one other patient so far. What follows is an account of how the next few weeks unfolded. Marit first began to notice a difference after around a week.

"It felt as if something in my hands relaxed," she says. After a while, she was able to walk down stairs normally—she no longer had to take them one by one. She tied her shoelaces herself; cut bread again. "Those are the kinds of things where you notice an improvement. I didn't go from being bedridden to jumping around the room, but I felt a little bit better every day," she says.

A couple of weeks after the first injection I wrote an email to Anders at Inven2. I told him that I got the results from the blood samples of Patient 2, and that she had been suffering from an extremely aggressive illness and had tried every treatment possible. "I initially didn't dare to include her as our second patient because of her destructive disease," I wrote.

Marit's blood tests were just as convincing as those for the first patient. Her CRP level reduced from forty-four to twenty-one. Another test we use to measure inflammation is erythrocyte sedimentation rate (ESR), and for Marit this was now equal to that of a healthy person. The effects I observed on the first two test patients were far more impressive than those I had seen in the study where we only administered the medication for five days. And Marit didn't stop there.

Marit was part of a group of eight friends who were planning a cycling trip in the spring of that year. Just a few weeks earlier it would have been unthinkable that Marit might have joined them, but she now felt her condition improving day by day. On the Friday they were set to leave, she stood at Tønsberg Station with her bicycle alongside the others. The weather was beautiful, and they set out toward Tjøme and Verdens Ende. Marit's friends were skeptical about how the trip might go, but Marit felt wonderful.

"It wasn't me who was trailing behind, at any rate—that's never been my style!" laughs Marit. I'll never forget the text message I received when she had returned home to Larvik. She had cycled nearly a hundred miles in just a few days.

"I think I was fitter than all the rest of them. In the end, they wondered whether they could have a bit of whatever I was taking! They couldn't believe it was true," she says.

It was only a little over a month since Marit had received her first dose of a GnRH inhibitor. This was a patient with whom the doctors had tried everything, with little success. Her condition had been up and down for years—but now she had just cycled farther and faster than any of her healthy friends.

"It was unreal," she says.

Her blood tests showed that her inflammation was almost gone.

I HAD NOW followed the amazing journeys of two patients over the course of just a few months. Jørund, Anders, and I discussed how we could take the results further.

"What about these hormones in men, how is it supposed to work on them?" Jørund asked at a meeting.

"You have testicles, don't you?" I joked. After all, it isn't only women who have sex hormones. But this was an important question. Would the medicine work on men? And might it also prove effective in treating other autoimmune diseases?

We needed a male test patient, and this was how I came to meet Jan. In 1941, the year Jan was born, the term "autoimmunity" didn't even exist. It took over forty years before someone could finally tell Jan why he had been so ill since childhood. His story illustrates just how tough life has been for many patients suffering from autoimmune diseases.

Only old people get rheumatism

I FIRST MET Jan in the corridor of Betanien Hospital. At the time he was worn out from a long period spent in very poor health, so it wasn't difficult to ask whether he would be interested in trying an experimental medicine. Jan answered that he would have agreed to cut off his hand if someone said it might make him better. At the time, it took him an hour to get out of bed in the morning, and the stairs to his first-floor apartment seemed like a Mount Everest.

"Imagine cutting off your legs and walking on the stumps— that's how it felt," he says today. After Jan had struggled out of bed with the help of his partner and finally made it to the chair on the veranda, he would stare down at his coffee cup with longing. He could no longer lift it.

Jan has been in and out of hospital for decades. He's seen treatments come and go, gulped down pills, and sat in the corridor on a drip. He was a patient at Betanien when the only available treatment was a huge pine hot tub.

"We'd lie there with the steaming water turning our bodies red, and two ladies topping it up with freshly boiled water whenever it cooled down," he says.

After living with his condition for over seventy years, Jan has regularly experienced setbacks and frustration in his encounters with the health service. This isn't uncommon for patients suffering from diseases many doctors don't know very much about. It still often takes a long time to get a diagnosis, and many patients describe being met with distrust by the very health service that is supposed to help get them through such crises. According to an American survey, almost half of all patients with autoimmune diseases have at some point been branded chronic complainers in their encounters with the health service. When doctors can't find clear answers through the usual examinations, it's easy to put the responsibility onto the patients themselves. Diagnosing a patient is often a long process, and all the while the patient lives in uncertainty. So what was wrong with Jan?

EVEN BACK WHEN Jan was a child, his parents understood that something was amiss. The five-year-old boy would try to keep up with the other children running down the street, but he would constantly stumble and fall. His legs failed. After his health check in second grade, the doctor sent Jan's mother and father a message.

"There's something wrong with Jan. His spine is completely crooked, but we don't know why," said the doctor. The staff at the local hospital confirmed the problem, but they too had no solution to the mystery. The young boy on the examination table was clearly in pain. They could hardly touch his lower back and the area around one of his hips. It seemed like a form of rheumatism, but the doctors weren't satisfied with this as an explanation.

"Only old people get rheumatism, so they thought it was impossible I might have it," says Jan.

Jan limped through his childhood on his useless legs in pain. Only when he was ten years old did he finally have an X-ray taken. The doctors stood before the light box and looked at the dark patches on the image that should have been white. Could the X-rays have been mixed up with some from the geriatric department? Jan's left hip was completely destroyed—at just ten years old. His mother and father had two options. Their son could either lie in the hospital on traction for a year—a form of round-the-clock, 365-day state-authorized torture. Or they could try to operate.

"It was almost unheard of to do a hip replacement on a child, but luckily that's what my parents decided to go for," says Jan.

After the Second World War, thousands of young Americans returned home from a European bloodbath. Many arms and legs were lost on the battlefield, and so a new area of research blossomed as never before—prostheses. Without the war, Jan would never have had a usable hip. The surgeons at the hospital were sent one of the new prostheses from the United States. Materials from the production of weapons were used to create a hip joint and thigh bone. When Jan woke from his operation, he had an American rocket in his hip.

The prosthesis helped, but Jan wasn't cured by it. The pain and stiffness came and went through better and worse periods, but they were never completely absent. He struggled through a physically demanding work life at the local shipyard, while his doctors continued to scratch their heads for another thirty years.

"When the doctors at the hospital look at you in a way that indicates they think you're lying, what are you supposed to do? When you can hardly get out of bed in the morning, but nobody believes you?" he says.

—⁂—

ONE DAY IN 1984, Jan was referred to a rheumatology specialist at Betanien Hospital. The doctor listened to Jan's story, bent, stretched, and squeezed his body, and studied X-rays of his back and hip. Then he said the magic words: "I know what's wrong with you."

Jan has ankylosing spondylitis—severe inflammation that primarily occurs in the joints of the spine, but when the disease arises in childhood it often attacks other large joints, such as the hips and knees. Many patients are able to function fairly normally, but some are severely affected. Although the cause of ankylosing spondylitis is unknown, we think an autoimmune reaction is involved. This is one of the most common autoimmune diseases. In Norway, it affects just under 1 percent of the population—around forty thousand people. This is one of the few examples of an autoimmune disease that prefers men.

Ankylosing spondylitis is also fond of northerners. If you come from the north of Norway, your risk of developing the disease is double that of people from the south of the country. The Sami, Indigenous people from the northern Nordic region, are at even greater risk. This is all down to genes. Almost all patients suffering from ankylosing spondylitis have the HLA-B27 gene. This is much more common among northerners than southerners, and most common among the Sami. In many African countries it is practically nonexistent.

But does this mean that the disease is worryingly hereditary? Well, it's not quite that simple. Ten percent of us have the HLA-B27 gene—far more than those who will actually develop the disease. Most individuals with this gene go through their lives without the cells of their immune systems ever caring about their spinal joints. This is yet another example of the cunning interplay between nature and nurture—here, too, it is a triggering environmental factor that will determine whether or not an individual will become ill.

For Jan, it was a relief to finally have an answer to his life's greatest question, even though by this point he was over forty years old. But the downside was that there was little treatment available. Physical activity is the most important factor in staying healthy, but Jan had done hard manual labor all his life and it clearly hadn't helped. In the years before I met him, Jan had tried various medicines without finding anything that worked. He was all out of options.

—ɱ—

I GAVE JAN the first dose of a GnRH inhibitor in the autumn of 2014. And just like the patients suffering from rheumatoid arthritis, he saw a change fairly quickly.

"I felt better, but I didn't dare trust it. I was afraid that I'd be disappointed in yet another medicine," says Jan today. Eventually he told me that something was changing. He was experiencing less pain, and his range of motion returned. Jan also has ulcerative colitis, a chronic inflammatory disease of the gut. This improved as well, and tests showed that his inflammation had significantly reduced.

"I've never had this kind of improvement from anything else," he told me. He was soon able to walk down the steps from his apartment to collect the newspaper again. He drove his car into town without problems. And on warm mornings on the veranda he lifted his coffee cup to his lips with a smile.

Did this mean that GnRH inhibitors might work on more than just rheumatoid arthritis? And also on men?

Expanding the tests

WE TESTED THE medication on more patients. Most of them had rheumatoid arthritis, but we also permitted some patients with ankylosing spondylitis, systemic sclerosis, and lupus to try the treatment. Some of them had secondary diagnoses in which inflammation was the main problem, such as psoriasis and inflammatory bowel disease, so we would be able to see if these symptoms improved too. We also collaborated with neurologists to test the medicine on multiple sclerosis patients. Only patients who had no other treatment alternatives were offered the medication.

A man with lupus made a particular impression on me. This inflammatory disease can affect the entire body and cause symptoms in many organs and areas. The most common are the skin, joints, kidneys, blood, and nervous system. *Lupus* is the Latin word for wolf. Several hundred years ago, the disease was given this name because it was believed that the classic rash on patients' faces was reminiscent of a wolf bite.

Nine out of ten lupus patients are women, but men who develop the disease are often severely affected. This man was attending the pain clinic at the hospital for help with his intense pain. He was also struggling to walk because the blood vessels in his feet were so inflamed.

Those suffering from lupus aren't exactly spoiled for choice when it comes to treatment alternatives. But among the more effective are medicines that are usually used to treat malaria. This is yet another example of a medical discovery that was made due to chance and vigilant researchers. During the Second World War, a number of battles were fought in the Pacific, and malaria was a problem for the Allied troops. Millions of soldiers were therefore given malaria medications. Some of them had rheumatic diseases such as lupus, and these soldiers reported that the medicine seemed to improve their symptoms. After the war, research proved that the soldiers were right. The medicines relieved the symptoms to a certain extent, and they remain some of the most used medications in the treatment of lupus today. Exactly why it works is a question researchers are still looking to answer, but the medications seem to suppress the immune system through various mechanisms.

Although many patients with lupus live long and happy lives, it can still be a potentially life-threatening disease. This man was suffering from a serious case of the illness. We were all out of options and believed it to be ethically justifiable to try treating him using a GnRH inhibitor.

After just a few months of treatment, the man booked a holiday to Poland and was able to walk normally again. With the medications usually used to treat lupus, we see that on average patients improve by around 60 percent after a year. With the GnRH inhibitor, this patient passed that point after just four weeks. Many lupus patients also have trouble with their kidneys—as did this fellow—but over the course of just a few weeks his kidney samples normalized. He had several nasty sores caused by the disease, too, which now gradually improved as well. Not only did the patient feel better, but his tests showed that his inflammation had reduced.

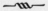

THE OTHER TEST patients also reported feeling better—some significantly, others just a little—and this was reflected in their blood tests. These were patients who no longer responded to the usual medicines—a group who are notoriously difficult to treat. The chance that anything would work for them was small. In an equivalent group of rheumatoid arthritis patients who were given anti-TNF, studies indicated that only around four in ten patients experienced any improvement.

I had before-and-after photos from my first test patient, Sandra. Before treatment her ankles were swollen and full of inflammation, but shortly after she started taking the GnRH inhibitor the swelling and inflammation was almost gone. I also started filming my patients, just as Ravinder Maini did when testing anti-TNF for the first time. Maini had to prove that what the doctors were seeing was real—and nothing is more convincing than video footage. I filmed my patients walking down the stairs before and after treatment. For many of them, the second video showed a huge improvement.

We were administering an experimental treatment; this wasn't a proper study, so we had to interpret the results with the utmost caution. But our test patients showed us that something was definitely at work—something it was important to get to the bottom of.

—⚯—

HOWEVER, THERE WAS still no progress with the pharmaceutical companies. Inven2 discussed my findings with several of them, but for various reasons none could be tempted to bite. I knew the staff at Inven2 were working hard, but I was still frustrated that things had reached a standstill. They must have found me quite irritating as I'd repeatedly call during evenings and holidays to ask them all kinds of questions. I called to bug them once again.

"We've tried, Anita. None of the major pharmaceutical companies are interested, so we just can't prioritize this," said the staff.

"Okay," I said. There wasn't much else to say.

I went out onto the balcony of my office. It was raining. The images of all my test patients swirled around in my head. For a brief moment I was back in Mum's bedroom in Liverpool; could hear her rhythmic breathing as she slept, which meant she would at least have a few hours free from the pain.

I wasn't ready to give up just yet.

15

THE BILLION-DOLLAR COMPANIES ARRIVE

*"Many in the field believe we are at the dawn of
a golden age which will see major benefits for patients
in the form of both treatments and cures."*

**FROM *60 YEARS OF IMMUNOLOGY*,
BRITISH SOCIETY FOR IMMUNOLOGY, 2016**

WAS THERE SOMETHING we were missing? We'd seen test patients throw out their crutches after just a few weeks. Others traveled long distances by bicycle after previously having struggled to get out of bed. We saw blood tests indicating that patients' inflammation had almost completely vanished. The potential market for a new medicine to treat inflammation is huge—millions of patients use cortisone, TNF inhibitors, and other anti-inflammatory medications daily. For a pharmaceutical company, it had to be worth investing a little money to find out whether GnRH inhibitors work. So why weren't any of them interested?

Inven2 had been in touch with their business contacts in the relevant companies, and we discussed whether a brief summary of our findings would be enough to convince them.

"We can't claim to treat a spectrum of autoimmune diseases with just a couple of pages of explanation," I said to Jørund and Anders. I understood the need to be brief and catchy in dealings with the business world, but it seemed unprofessional to send out a short note stating that we might be able to treat rheumatoid arthritis, MS, psoriasis, and a number of other things. Who would believe us?

Once again, I sought Andrew Schally's advice, sending an email to him and his right-hand man at the lab in Miami, Norman Block. I attached a brief explanation, together with the videos of the test patients.

"I hope you agree there is potential. I do believe many patients could be helped," I wrote, and asked whether they had any suggestions as to who I might contact within the pharmaceutical industry. It was a Friday, and the weekend was fast approaching, so I sent off the email and thought little more about it.

But Monday morning took an unexpected turn. Block forwarded the email to an acquaintance, one of the senior managers in Ferring Pharmaceuticals. Ferring owned the rights to one of the medications we had used.

"Take a look at the video—very impressive," Block wrote to his contact.

Just a few hours later, the manager responded. "I am intrigued by Dr. Kåss's research," he started, explaining that this was an opportunity he had never considered before. "I will obviously need to broaden my thinking!" he wrote, and politely asked whether he could share the email with his colleagues within the company.

In just a couple of days, things were suddenly underway. Ferring was definitely interested, and the company invited us to a meeting at its headquarters in Copenhagen.

ALONG THE WAY, I'd learned something very important: to be sure to contact the actual decision makers within the organizations. And the video footage was crucial—it enabled people to see the patients' improvements with their own eyes.

I scoured the web for the email addresses of senior managers within the major pharmaceutical companies—some of them were extremely well hidden. Sometimes I could spend an entire day hunting down just a single email address. I wrote a sixteen-page summary and formulated a new email message. The people to whom I was directing my inquiry were specialists—they needed a thorough explanation of my findings, not just a summary in one or two pages. I inserted links to videos of the test patients, both before and after treatment. And then I started to send out my queries.

Pharmaceutical giant Pfizer was the first company I contacted— it was like sending an unsolicited email to the CEO of Coca-Cola and hoping for a response. I took a deep breath and clicked "Send." That was that, I told myself, and returned to my daily tasks thinking that it would be at least a couple of weeks before I received an answer—if I received any response at all.

It took twenty-five minutes. Pfizer requested more information.

Over the next few weeks I worked my way down the list, sending emails to the managing and medical directors of AbbVie, AstraZeneca, and MSD, among others—all companies with a relevant medication in their portfolio. "I hope you'll agree that there is significant untapped potential for GnRH inhibitors," I concluded my email. Every company I contacted responded—and not only with polite empty phrases. Several of them were genuinely interested. I now knew that this might actually work—that we could do it.

"Woohoo!" I wrote to Jørund and Anders when one of the larger companies requested a meeting. Our energy had returned, and things were finally happening. We started to believe again.

The sun was shining. I went out into the park behind the hospital and lay on my back beside the statue of a local polar explorer. My lab coat became a snow angel in the grass. I lay there like that for several minutes, just to enjoy the feeling.

Relief

MANY LENGTHY EMAIL exchanges with the pharmaceutical giants now awaited me, and the process was a rollercoaster ride. But one company—Ferring—stood out. The company was started in Sweden by a German researcher fleeing the Nazis between the wars and is still owned by the same family today. The company's founder died some years ago, but on their website I read his advice to young researchers: "It's better to work on research without thinking about money. Goal-oriented research is remarkably unproductive." This was a company that shared my values. Jørund, Anders, and I set out for their headquarters in Copenhagen.

Ferring's high-rise office premises are situated just a short taxi ride from Kastrup airport, where they tower tall and lonely above Ørestad train station. At the top of the building, the blue letters of the company's name assert their authority. We waited in reception, all of us silent. Jørund switched off completely, as if suddenly struck by the gravity of the situation. He fished out his cell phone and started to play a game of chess, perhaps psyching himself up for possible objections and critical questions. I tried to appear unfazed at suddenly finding myself and my research in such a position.

The meeting room was on the top floor, and Ferring had put one of their most senior members of staff on the case. He was snobby in a charming sort of way, a bit like James Bond. Later, Jørund warned me not to fall for his charm.

"He knows that all you're interested in is a bigger study; that you don't care about the money," he said.

We sat around the conference table. It was time to convince the company that we had something worth listening to. As the meeting progressed, I noticed that the tone in the representative's voice changed from skeptical to curious. *This is actually going well*, I thought to myself.

"We're open to doing a study on this," the representative from Ferring said finally. I did my best to keep a straight face. We were close. Very close.

As we left the building, Jørund and Anders were enthusiastic— I had no idea what was normal at such meetings, but I knew that something good had happened and let myself be carried along by their excitement. I glanced back over my shoulder, toward the dark facade.

"We probably shouldn't look so ecstatic, right under their noses," I said.

"Right," said Jørund, and we all bundled into a taxi.

At the airport, we raised a glass and toasted our successful meeting, all of us relieved and happy. "Smile!" said Jørund. He was sure we had it in the bag. "Anita—you're going to be rich!" he joked, the world's biggest grin plastered across his face. I couldn't help but laugh.

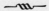

NEGOTIATIONS TAKE TIME, and I'm an impatient person. In the spring of 2015 I took yet another look down the list of relevant pharmaceutical companies and stopped at Astellas Pharma. The company was developing a GnRH inhibitor in tablet form. They were worth a try.

I formulated a new email of the type I was by now well practiced at writing. "I hope you'll agree that there is significant untapped potential for GnRH inhibitors," I concluded the message before sending it off to the company.

Astellas's headquarters are situated in Tokyo, Japan. Despite not being as widely known as Pfizer, Merck, and Bayer, the company is estimated as being worth over US$20 billion. Astellas was developing a drug called ASP1707 for the treatment of prostate cancer. I suggested that they should test it for the treatment of rheumatoid arthritis.

Just a few days after sending the email I received a polite response requesting more information, and over the following days the Japanese indicated that they were ready for action. One of the company's managers sent a personal reply to my email, hoping that we could have "a productive discussion on a potential collaboration." Jørund was excited at the prospect of another proposal. "We have to go to Japan!" he said. "And make sure we take a nicely wrapped gift with us," he added with a smile. We were suddenly in negotiations with two different companies.

The Japanese were serious and left nothing to chance—they wanted to know every last detail about the studies I'd carried out. There was definitely something in the air. Now it was just a question of which company would close the deal.

Money problems

THE DISCUSSIONS WITH the pharmaceutical companies dragged on, and the months went by. I would soon be out of funding, and the chances of undertaking more research were starting to look slim. Unless things changed soon, I'd have to go back to working as a doctor. The director of Betanien Hospital was aware that money had become a problem.

"What will you do if you can't get hold of more research funding?" he asked me one day.

It wasn't a difficult question to answer.

"I'm going to keep banging on doors. Again and again and again," I said.

But I was worried. I was running the risk of leaving the entire project high and dry. Might it be possible to find funding outside the traditional channels? We contacted the Telemark Development Fund—a fund established from the profits of the hydropower industry, which supported local projects.

"I understand the problem—I'll see what we can do," said the fund manager. He was efficient and arranged a meeting with possible sources of support from the surrounding area.

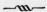

ON THE DAY of the meeting I was late and so hurried toward the blue-gray concrete block of a building in Skien city center. It was pouring rain, and I splashed through the puddles in my high-heeled shoes as I passed the factory chimney from the industry that had once dominated the little island.

Inside, the others who had been invited to the meeting were already seated around a large conference table. "Hi, Anita," said Jørund, getting up from his chair. He had the face of a businessman used to keeping calm under pressure. "Relax. Here, have a coffee," he said, pouring me a cup. It was embarrassing to be late—especially as I was usually always half an hour early. There was a lot on the line. This might be our last chance to secure project financing.

I opened my laptop, glancing at my fingers as I did so. Red nail polish had seemed like a bad idea, and so I'd stopped off at the supermarket on the way to buy some nail polish remover. In the car I'd scrubbed away the color, and I now stank of the strong chemical. Could it get any worse? I looked up at the group and smiled. A posh British accent wasn't going to do much good here.

"Thank you all for coming," I said, and received a few nods in return. I introduced myself and the project and explained why further research was important. "We're looking to land a global deal with a pharmaceutical company," I said in conclusion—a big claim coming from an unknown researcher at a little hospital in Skien. But we sold ourselves as best we could.

Jørund and I left the meeting together. We'd long discussed what was required to take the research a step further. The problem with GnRH inhibitors is that they also act as a form of chemical castration—which for young patients is particularly unfavorable. There is always uncertainty surrounding the long-term use of medications, and so far studies had only followed the use of GnRH inhibitors for up to five years. We therefore had no idea whether treatment over a longer period of time would lead to as-yet-unknown side effects. With greater knowledge comes new ideas, and I started to mull over a question that came to intrigue me more and more. Was it possible to create a medication that worked just as effectively, but without chemically castrating the patients?

GnRH doesn't just act locally in the brain—it is also able to bind to several of the body's immune cells directly. Some immune cells are even able to produce and extract GnRH themselves. The hormone is therefore also found outside the closed system of the brain, and in my mind this could mean only one thing: the hormone was of wider significance than its role in the chain reaction that produces sex hormones. It worked directly on the immune cells. Was that why it seemed to have an effect on the inflammatory response? Perhaps treatment wasn't about blocking the sex hormones. Instead, maybe it was about preventing GnRH from binding with the immune cells. The idea was to create a medication that could block the hormone outside the brain—so the sex hormones could roam free.

Before we went our separate ways in the rain, Jørund took hold of my shoulder.

"Do the lab tests that need to be done to move another step forward," he said.

"And who's going to do that?" I asked, staring uncomprehendingly at him.

"You," Jørund said.

"How am I going to do it? I hardly know where the 'on' button on half the lab equipment is!" I said, laughing.

"You'll figure it out," he said.

Just a few weeks later we received our decision from the meeting participants—they would provide us with 2 million kroner, or about US$200,000. A short while later, we also received funding from the Research Council of Norway. I could breathe a sigh of relief.

Now all I needed was a laboratory.

The lab in the storeroom

I NEEDED SOMEWHERE I'd be able to work alone, day and night. I would have to learn how to use advanced lab equipment, and so went on YouTube and worked my way through instructional videos and ABCs for lab machines. Of course, I was doomed to make a fool of myself on the first few attempts—and would prefer to be able to do so without looking like the world's biggest buffoon in front of other researchers.

I checked whether it would be possible to set up a provisional lab at Betanien Hospital. The equipment I needed would cost a fortune, so it wasn't an option to buy everything outright, but I found a loophole—the companies rented out their equipment for a trial period, allowing people to test it before possibly making a purchase. Just a few telephone conversations were enough—I suddenly had all the equipment I needed. All I had to do was remember to send it back when the trial period came to an end.

Great, I thought—now all I needed was a room in which I could set everything up. On the second floor of the hospital was an old storage room with no windows. It would have to do. I made sure that conditions were sterile and set everything up as best as I could. Now that the practical side of things was up and running there was only one thing missing—sufficient knowledge of chemistry.

A GnRH inhibitor is an artificial form of GnRH. The medication binds to the receptors on the cells, much like a key that fits inside a lock. But despite the key fitting in the keyhole, it has no function and can't be turned—the door therefore remains closed, and the GnRH doesn't work. In order to create a GnRH inhibitor, I would have to replace small parts of the hormone with something else, and to do this I would need to know the chemical structure of the hormone. I was no chemist, but I could read. And so I purchased five medical chemistry textbooks and started to learn how I should approach my task.

Luckily, GnRH is a relatively simple hormone, and it was therefore possible to find out what kinds of structures might have potential as a new medicine. I worked extremely hard in yet another field within which I had little prior knowledge. It was often simply a case of trial and error. Eventually, I received assistance from a doctor from India and a bioengineer from Sri Lanka. Both of them were receiving social benefits and needed on-the-job training—and I needed help.

We stood in the poky storeroom for days and nights on end. A huge hole in the wall had been patched up with gray cinder blocks, and cardboard boxes full of equipment were stacked on the blue shelves. On the walls, we hung notes detailing how things should be done. After months of trying, we finally discovered how we could test the various substances that might prove suitable medicines. We purchased immune cells from patients with rheumatoid arthritis and studied how the various substances affected them.

It was manual work and extremely labor intensive—but also absolutely possible once we understood how.

Other scientists might be lucky enough to be offered lab space, the latest equipment, and assistants on a silver platter—and I must admit that I often envied them as I stood in the stuffy, windowless storage room in the middle of the night. But at the same time, it was a special feeling, doing everything from scratch. I was on a voyage of discovery.

—ᴍ—

ON CHRISTMAS EVE of 2015 I received a message on my phone. It was from Jørund.

"Merry Christmas, Anita! Be sure to check your email once more before new year :)."

The email said that one of the companies had made a decision. They wanted to make a deal.

"It's a deal"

IN APRIL, I received another text message. Jørund and Anders wanted to give me and the director of the hospital an update on the negotiations. I could tell that it was good news. We sat down in front of the computer screen in the director's office and soon made contact with Jørund and Anders via Skype.

"It's a deal with Astellas," said Jørund.

I looked at the director—he was struggling to maintain his professional expression. I leaned over and kissed him on the cheek, making both of us relax and burst out laughing. We signed the contract that summer—the deal was finally done.

The money involved in such agreements is often overhyped, and this was certainly the case for us. But everything depends on the medicine actually being proved effective through further research. A small sum is received upon signing the contract—the money will only start to trickle in if the company takes new steps toward approval of the drug. In order to sell the medication for the treatment of rheumatoid arthritis, Astellas would have to carry out several studies to see whether it actually worked.

If all this proves successful, the potential earnings comprise tens of millions of US dollars. Overall, our deal was the largest license agreement between a hospital and a pharmaceutical company ever to be signed in Norwegian history.

I WAS RELIEVED to finally have a deal wrapped up, but I also felt uneasy. It was important that the next stages of the research be undertaken properly and with care—and not least, I wanted to stay involved. I was, after all, the only person in the world with experience in using GnRH inhibitors in the treatment of auto-immune diseases. But the Japanese wanted to take the next steps on their own. My further involvement was sacrificed at the negotiating table.

Research and business are two different planets. During these hectic years, I sometimes felt as if my research was nothing but a commodity—that concern for the patients was shoved to the background. The main concern should be to ensure that further research can succeed, but I was excluded from these important discussions. I had brought the research all this way almost single-handedly, but that no longer seemed to count for anything.

I'm sure many researchers have experienced the discomfort of losing control of their work when their findings suddenly become business ventures. I feared that people would fail to take good care of the research baby I had given birth to and raised over the past several years.

But by now, the grapevine was also in full swing. Emails from desperate patients wanting to try a GnRH inhibitor rapidly accumulated in my inbox. They had tried everything, but now they had new hope.

"Please consider me as a volunteer," one wrote. "This is a cry in the dark," wrote another, begging for any advice that might help his wife. A woman in her fifties told me she had been living with rheumatoid arthritis since she was six years old. "Since I was small I've hoped and believed that one fine day, a medicine that can give me a better life will be discovered. I'm still hoping," she wrote.

These patients deserved a larger study that would clarify whether GnRH inhibitors actually work. That's what was really on the line—people's lives. Everything to do with money and patents mustn't result in patients losing opportunities and hope. Of course I knew that the companies needed to earn money, that they wanted exclusive deals to protect themselves from the competition. That's how the system works. But would it help the hundreds of patients who had sent me desperate emails?

In early 2017, the media broke the news of the deal with Astellas. And once again, my life changed overnight.

16

NOTHING IS BLACK AND WHITE

*"We must adjust to changing times and
still hold to unchanging principles."*
FORMER US PRESIDENT JIMMY CARTER,
QUOTING HIS HIGH SCHOOL TEACHER
JULIA COLEMAN, IN HIS INAUGURAL ADDRESS, 1977

I WOKE UP TO a text message from a friend: "You're on the front page of the *Finansavisen!*" I sat up in bed and did a quick online search—and there was my face, plastered across the front page of the largest Norwegian financial newspaper. The headline was "The biggest license deal of our time," followed by "Anita Kåss discovers pill for rheumatoid arthritis." The story spread rapidly throughout the Norwegian media. "Her medicine gives patients a new life," wrote the public broadcaster NRK. In the country's biggest newspaper, VG, the headline was "Doctor Anita Kåss develops new medicine." "This is the biggest license agreement ever to be entered into by a Norwegian hospital," said the CEO of Inven2 via each and every media channel.

The pressure from journalists and others wishing to speak to me was greater than I ever could have imagined. I was inundated with phone calls—it was impossible to answer them all. Robin acted as my secretary, separating out what was urgent from what could wait.

The reception staff at the hospital told me that someone from *Skavlan* had been trying to get hold of me—they had asked that I call them back. *Skavlan? It must be a local newspaper or small magazine,* I thought. It wasn't until a couple of days later that I remembered to return their call. Only then did I understand that this was hardly some obscure publication.

"Um... Do you mean *Skavlan* as in the TV show?" I finally asked. In the midst of all the chaos I hadn't realized that it was Scandinavia's biggest talk show that was trying to get hold of me.

There was a brief silence on the other end of the line. I can just imagine how the journalist must have chuckled to himself, glancing at his colleagues; pointing to the telephone and rolling his eyes.

"Yes, this is *Skavlan*—as in the TV show."

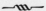

AND SO THAT'S how I ended up in Stockholm just a short time later, sitting in the talk show's greenroom and waiting to go on stage. On the screen, I could see the host talking to the head of the Swedish Academy—the institution that awards the Nobel Prizes. Just a few months earlier they had announced that the winner of the Nobel Prize in Literature for 2016 was Bob Dylan. When I finally took a seat in the chair opposite the talk show host, my voice was shaky.

"Congratulations," he said, smiling. "Why did researching rheumatoid arthritis become so important to you?"

I nodded cautiously. "My mother had rheumatoid arthritis," I said. "Sadly, she died of it when I was thirteen years old." In an instant, my personal story had become public property.

I can feel the reverberations from those few minutes on the talk show to this day. I was immediately inundated with emails; hand-written letters began to pile up at the office. Hundreds of patients desperate for relief. I developed a gnawing guilt at the fact that I couldn't respond to all of them—it was an impossible task. Even now, I continue to receive inquiries from patients almost daily.

When you've appeared on TV, you suddenly have the unbounded trust of countless strangers. The media has an immense power to build you up, but it can just as easily knock you down. Luckily, I've so far only experienced the former.

What if it's wrong?

WHAT IF FURTHER research shows that GnRH inhibitors don't work? This is an outcome I'm prepared for. Science has its own evolution; research is change. What is true today might not be true tomorrow. The history of scientific research is full of promis-ing findings that later fall apart, and the same thing might happen with my research. I believe that what I've discovered could turn out to be important, and that it might give patients a better life. But I'm also aware that it might be wrong. As I said in an interview with NRK: "There are no guarantees. If you knew how the results were going to turn out, there'd be no need to do the research."

The medication Astellas is testing is under development. It's a GnRH inhibitor, but it's not the same medicine as the one we used in our trials. Small differences between medications can lead to significantly different results. If Astellas's medicine doesn't work, that doesn't mean the story will end there. It will just mean that we need to do more research; dig deeper.

If at the end of the day further research shows that the medication doesn't work, this will of course be a huge disappointment—but that's only fitting. If I don't succeed, that *should* mean something to me.

The hope is that this medication will provide a new treatment for severe inflammation—something that will have a greater effect than the treatments currently available, and that will have fewer side effects. If so, this will be a breakthrough for the many diseases in which inflammation is the main problem. It won't be a cure, but it might dampen the flames enough for patients to be able to live normal lives.

I've seen patients hobble into my office, their bodies bent and crooked, only to throw away their crutches or cycle hundreds of miles after just a few weeks. I've seen ulcers vanish. I've seen inflammation disappear from blood tests. I've heard Marit tell me about "a whole new world," and Jan say that "it was like entering the kingdom of heaven."

What I observe in my patients, and what they tell me, is most important. If something is having a positive effect, we have to find out what that is. It might be able to give people a better life. And for some patients, it might be the only thing able to give them any kind of life at all.

—⚶—

EVERY NOW AND AGAIN I dream about my mum. These dreams are always in black and white, and in them Mum is very ill, just as I remember her. But then one night I suddenly dreamed in color. In my dream, Mum was better. She was still unable to walk, but her condition had improved. I'd never dreamed about my mum getting better before.

I think that means that I'm doing something right. That my mum is proud of me. One day, I hope to wake from a dream in which she's healthy again.

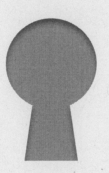

EPILOGUE:
THE SEARCH FOR
A LONGER LIFE

W E ARE BORN, and from then on life moves in only one direction—toward death. The body slowly ages. the skin changes, becomes looser, and we get wrinkles. Our bones become more porous. If we fall, we might break our wrist or hip—something that would never have happened in our youth. Our blood vessels change, becoming less elastic, weakening, and in some areas becoming lined with fat—we suffer strokes and heart attacks. Our hair turns gray, or white, or falls out. All this is easy to see. But what about the immune system? How does it change with age?

Where the immune system is concerned, it's wrong to say that the curve follows a continual downward trend. On the contrary, it goes quickly upward toward puberty, as the immune system grows stronger, before finally reaching its peak. The curve then flattens out for several years, and the body lives well with the army it has established during the first two decades of life. But eventually, things take a downward turn. For women, there is a shift during menopause, when the immune system takes a sudden hit. Once menopause is over, the aging process continues at a calmer pace.

Our defenses are divided into the innate immune system and the adaptive or acquired immune system. The cells of the innate immune system are already in place when we are born, but put on pause to avoid harmful attacks when we're still in our mother's womb. When a child makes its way out into the world, it's as if someone pushes the start button. After a fairly short period of time, the innate immune system—our home guard—is on full alert.

The acquired immune system, which consists of the body's special forces, needs time to be properly trained. We are therefore more susceptible to infection during the first years of life. There's a reason that childhood mortality is high in societies lacking adequate nutrition, hygiene, and vaccination programs. The special forces are programmed to fight all dangerous intruders that force their way into the body, but they require experience of combat.

When the special forces meet their nemesis and go to war, they are the perfect weapon. If they've done battle with an enemy before, these soldiers will remember him forever. Should a bacterium or virus attempt a new attack, the special forces are so well trained that they knock out the intruder before he's even managed to get a foot in the door—we'll never suffer from chicken pox twice, for example. In the event of a second infection, the special forces are mercilessly effective and destroy the virus before it manages to cause trouble.

The memories of these special forces form the foundation of what may be medical research's most important discovery—vaccines. As children, we are vaccinated against the measles, mumps, and rubella. We're injected with a weakened version of each virus, which isn't harmful but is sufficient to give the special forces the training they need. If any of the viruses should attack at a later date, the immune system is so effective that we won't become ill.

Childhood and adolescence are one long period of training for the immune system. Because we all experience different infections and challenges in life, we each develop an immune system that is unique. Even identical twins have their own individual armed forces.

The defenses we build up function perfectly for a long time, but at a certain point our armed forces get tired. The soldiers age, and some of them handle this more poorly than others. Inflammation increases, which can then increase the risk of cardiovascular diseases. Infections are met with less resistance, and when we become ill it takes longer for us to recover. Every year, many elderly people die of a flu virus that would have been completely harmless to them at a younger age. An increased risk of cancer goes hand in hand with a weakened immune system, as our immune cells work to keep this kind of uncontrolled cell division in check throughout our lives.

The cells of our immune system also become more confused, and the risk of developing autoimmune diseases increases. The entire system becomes more and more autoimmune. It's as if the armed forces within us say that they've had enough—it's time for them to be discharged.

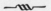

THE AGING OF the immune system is our countdown—it's the reason we die. Some believe that this immune weakness is the price we pay for living on borrowed time. In recent centuries, our life expectancy has dramatically increased. The body is unable to keep up. In an evolutionary sense, we are only of value while we're able to have children. Our immune system must keep us alive as young adults so that we can pass on our genes.

The most striking example of this aging is seen in the tiny organ called the thymus. This is where the T cells' military academy is located. The organ is crucial for these vital special forces. The thymus looks like a butterfly, situated directly behind the breastbone, squeezed in between the lungs. It grows until we reach puberty, when it reaches the size of a thumb. Then something unnerving happens. Slowly but surely, the thymus shrinks. This is one of the main reasons the immune system functions less effectively as we get older, but why this happens, we don't know.

One of the leading theories is that it's all down to energy. Keeping the military academy in the thymus going is a demanding task. After having trained special forces for several decades and building up solid defenses, perhaps the body just thinks it's done enough. It needs to use its available energy elsewhere—an aging body requires much more maintenance and waste handling, for example. Interestingly enough, the thymus also shrinks temporarily during pregnancy; the same thing happens in people who fast. The body has to use its limited energy resources on more important things.

The hormone GnRH also appears to play a role here. Researchers have stimulated GnRH production in rats and observed that the thymus grows. Is it possible that this hormone affects the aging of the immune system?

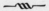

THE IMMUNE SYSTEM is born, then grows and increases in strength before it slowly withers into old age, just like the rest of the body. If an aging immune system is the reason we become ill and die, might the fountain of youth also be found here? If there's one thing each and every one of us is striving for, including medical researchers, it's this—to live longer and healthier lives. We want to surmount the limits nature has set for us. Might it be possible to slow the aging process by keeping the immune system young?

One of the most marked changes that occurs when we get older is that the body enters a state of mild inflammation. If we could safely prevent this, perhaps we could also stay younger for longer. The medications currently available cause too many undesirable side effects to make them worth using—they do more harm than good. But what if we discover something else?

The ability to bear children is closely linked to the immune system. The sex hormones control reproduction, and GnRH is the master hormone that keeps the human race from extinction. Might the secret of a longer life lie in the hormone that creates new life? Of course this is pure speculation—but it's a beautiful thought.

Time to get back to the laboratory.

ACKNOWLEDGMENTS

T HE AUTHORS WOULD like to thank everyone at Cappelen Damm for their work on this book. Special thanks are due to our editor, Mari Bjørkeng, who provided thorough feedback and excellent follow-up throughout the process. We would also like to thank the Fritt Ord Foundation and the Norwegian Non-Fiction Writers and Translators Association for their belief in the project and for granting it financial support. Not least, we would like to thank all the patients who have contributed their stories—especially Marit and Jan.

Anita Kåss would like to thank Robin and his family—Ingrid, Astrid, Hilde, and Peter. You have all been a huge source of support for me and my work. Robin's support also helped give me the courage to embark on this research.

Throughout the year I spent working on this book, Geir Arnfinn has been an important source of support. The same is true of several close friends who continually remind me that life is about more than just work. Thank you for being there for me.

Publishing this book has given me the opportunity to tell my story in my own words. This is an honest account of how I remember the events of recent years, but a story drawn from life has no single correct version—it is woven together from the differing experiences of different people. Some of the people in this story might perceive certain things differently from the way in which I remember them.

It is important for me to say that I greatly appreciate all the help I have received from everyone involved in my research, especially my colleagues and the management at Betanien Hospital, as well as Jørund and Anders at Inven2. I could never have done it without you. I would also like to extend my deepest gratitude to all the patients who have participated in my studies and supported my work.

Most important of all are my daughters—Dea, Maia, and Ingrid Marie. Their unconditional love has always given me strength.

Jørgen Jelstad would like to thank his employer, the journal *Utdanning*, and especially editor Knut Hovland, for the flexibility that has made work on this book possible. A huge thank-you to my close friend Erik Abild, who took the time to provide detailed feedback at an important stage in the writing process—it meant more to me than you know. Most of all, I would like to thank Lindis and Ravn. You make the world a better place in which to live, play, learn, and laugh.

OVERVIEW OF
AUTOIMMUNE DISEASES

T HIS IS AN attempt to provide an overview of the main diseases in which autoimmunity is thought to play a central role. Whether a specific condition is regarded as an autoimmune disease is a question of definition, and there are few diseases for which the main cause has been finally determined to be autoimmunity. Many are classified under terms such as immunological diseases, inflammatory diseases, or other umbrella terms.

How this list has been prepared

ONLY A FEW attempts have been made to create an overview of autoimmune diseases. Ours is based on the following:

- "Updated Assessment of the Prevalence, Spectrum and Case Definition of Autoimmune Disease," S. M. Hayter et al., *Autoimmunity Reviews*, 2012. This article lists 81 diagnoses.

- The American Autoimmune Related Diseases Association is a nonprofit organization that provides information and promotes research. They have a list containing 152 diagnoses.

- The Autoimmune Registry is a nonprofit organization that gathers statistics and information in a database for patients. They have a list of 155 diagnoses.

- Wikipedia has a "List of autoimmune diseases." As of June 2018, this consists of 145 diagnoses.

We have collated all the diagnoses and checked them against reliable sources before performing a subjective assessment as to whether or not they should be included. Some of the headings in this list are for groups of diseases that cover several diagnoses.

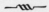

WE HAVE USED the following sources:

- *Norsk elektronisk legehåndbok* [Norwegian Online Medical Handbook] / Norsk helseinformatikk [Norwegian Health Informatics (database)] (nhi.no)

- BMJ Best Practice

- Medscape

- Uptodate.com

- Genetic and Rare Diseases Information Center/National Institutes of Health (NIH)

- American College of Rheumatology

Where we have also used additional sources, these are given under the relevant diagnosis.

Acquired angioedema (AAE)

WHAT IS IT? Inflammation in the small blood vessels of the dermis and mucous membranes leads to episodes of swelling in the face or body. The airways may also swell, which may be life-threatening. There are two types: type 1 is linked to lymphoma or autoimmune diseases, while type 2 is an autoimmune reaction against a protein in the blood. In cases of severe breathing difficulties, intubation may be necessary.

DID YOU KNOW? Angioedema is a common condition that often occurs in connection with hives (urticaria), but the autoimmune variant is extremely rare. As a general rule, angioedema is caused by an allergic reaction, such as to medications.

Acquired hemophilia

WHAT IS IT? Hemophilia is a bleeding disease, in which the blood fails to coagulate. Hemophilia may be inherited as a genetic disease, but the acquired variant is an autoimmune attack on an important part of the coagulation system. The patient often experiences bleeding in the skin, muscles, and mucous membranes. The mortality rate is 8–22 percent, but this must be viewed in light of the fact that it is often the elderly who are affected.

DID YOU KNOW? In a number of cases (2–11 percent) the disease seems to be triggered by pregnancy.

Acute disseminated encephalomyelitis (ADEM)

WHAT IS IT? The immune system attacks the insulation surrounding the neural pathways in the brain and spinal cord, resulting in inflammation. The same thing happens in multiple sclerosis, but while MS is chronic, ADEM almost always subsides after a brief attack. The disease occurs directly after an infection. Eight out of every ten patients are children under the age of ten. The symptoms worsen over the first few days and may finally result in paralysis and coma. Most of those affected recover, even in extreme cases. The disease is fatal for less than 2 percent of patients.

DID YOU KNOW? Children who have suffered from ADEM have a slightly increased risk of developing MS later in life.

Addison's disease

WHAT IS IT? Production of the adrenocortical hormones, including cortisol, fails. In the majority of patients, the cause is an autoimmune attack within the adrenal cortex. The condition is life-threatening, but with hormone replacement the prognosis is good. The disease may start with acute adrenal failure, an Addison's crisis. This can result in shock with a drop in blood pressure, dehydration, and lack of oxygen, and requires immediate treatment.

DID YOU KNOW? British doctor Thomas Addison first described the disease in 1855. Before the age of antibiotics, tuberculosis was the most important factor in adrenal failure.

EXTRA SOURCE: "Primær binyrebarksvikt—årsaker, diagnostikk og behandling," [Primary adrenal insufficiency causes, diagnostics and treatment] K. Løvås et al., *Journal of the Norwegian Medical Association*, 2005.

Alopecia areata

WHAT IS IT? The immune system seems to attack the hair follicles so that the hair falls out in clumps. It often starts on the head, and for men it often affects the facial hair. Some of those affected lose their eyebrows and the hair on their arms and legs. This is a common condition that affects up to 2 percent of the population. Over half of those affected recover within a year. Less than 10 percent develop the serious, chronic form.

DID YOU KNOW? Around 1 percent of those affected develop alopecia universalis and lose all their body hair.

Ankylosing spondylitis

WHAT IS IT? The immune system attacks the joints, resulting in inflammation, often in areas where tendons attach to bone. Affects the back, pelvis, and chest, and may also attack the shoulders, hips, and knees. Over 90 percent of those affected have a tissue type known as HLA-B27. If you have a parent with ankylosing spondylitis, there is a 15–20 percent chance that you will also be affected. Most patients function well; some experience hardly any symptoms. But some are affected so severely that they become disabled. Affects 0.1–1 percent of the population (with significant geographical variation) and is one of the most common autoimmune diseases.

DID YOU KNOW? Several famous people have spoken about what it's like to live with ankylosing spondylitis, including the singer of the band Imagine Dragons, Dan Reynolds, and the Secretary General of NATO, Jens Stoltenberg.

Anti-NMDA receptor encephalitis

WHAT IS IT? NMDA stands for N-methyl D-aspartate, a substance that activates a receptor in the brain. The immune system attacks the receptors, which results in brain inflammation (encephalitis). In around half of those affected, a tumor with tissue similar to the NMDA receptors may be the cause. Symptoms may develop, from flu-like symptoms to psychiatric symptoms such as delusions, hallucinations, and seizures. May finally result in breathing difficulties and coma. Most patients dramatically improve; many recover completely. Some experience serious aftereffects; few die.

DID YOU KNOW? The disease took the life of world-famous polar bear Knut. In 2011, the polar bear suffered a major seizure and drowned in a pool at Berlin's zoo in front of hundreds of shocked visitors. This was the first time the disease had been observed in animals.

EXTRA SOURCES:

1. "Anti-NMDA-Reseptorencefalitt," [Anti-NMDA receptor encephalitis] K. Engen et al., *Journal of the Norwegian Medical Association*, 2016.
2. "Knut Polar Bear Death Riddle Solved," Jonathan Amos, BBC News, August 27, 2015.

Antiphospholipid syndrome

WHAT IS IT? The immune system attacks the blood, which affects its ability to coagulate and causes it to clot more easily. This may result in an increased propensity for blood clots and/or repeated miscarriages. One to five percent of the population have the antibodies that cause the disease, but extremely few experience complications. Patients often have other autoimmune diseases in addition, such as SLE (lupus). Treatment involves preventing and treating blood clots using medications that thin the blood.

DID YOU KNOW? Less than 1 percent of those with this condition experience what is known as catastrophic antiphospholipid syndrome, which causes a number of blood clots over a short period of time and the failure of several of the body's organs. Around half of these patients die.

Antisynthetase syndrome

WHAT IS IT? The immune system attacks specific enzymes in the body, which can result in inflammation of the lungs, muscles, and joints. The symptoms vary depending on the tissue that is attacked. The prognosis varies, but many patients find that the disease disappears. However, recurrences are common. Whether and how severely the lungs are attacked is important for the patient's prognosis. Some patients die of lung failure.

DID YOU KNOW? The most common antibody in the disease is named after the patient in which researchers discovered it for the first time in 1980. The patient's name was John, and the antibody was therefore named Anti-Jo-1.

EXTRA SOURCE: "Antisyntetasesyndrom," [Antisynthetase syndrome] J. T. Gran, *Journal of the Norwegian Medical Association*, 2002.

Aplastic anemia

WHAT IS IT? A deficiency in blood cell production, which results in a low blood count (anemia). Research indicates that autoimmunity is the cause. Since the stem cells are affected, the body produces fewer blood cells of all types—red, white, and platelets. This results in symptoms such as fatigue, labored breathing, heart palpitations, and an increased risk of hemorrhage and infection. In younger patients bone marrow transplantation may be recommended, and 60–70 percent are then cured. Without treatment, the disease is fatal.

DID YOU KNOW? This is an extremely rare condition, which most often arises as a complication following intensive cancer treatment.

Autoimmune atrophic gastritis / pernicious anemia

WHAT IS IT? Gastritis is inflammation of the stomach lining, also known as gastric catarrh. In most cases, chronic gastritis is caused by the bacteria *Helicobacter pylori*, but it may also occur following an autoimmune attack on the parietal cells of the stomach.

These cells produce a protein that is important in the absorption of vitamin B_{12}. B_{12} deficiency can result in pernicious anemia—low blood count—which is fatal without treatment, and which may also cause nerve damage. Patients require lifelong treatment with vitamin B_{12} and iron. Pernicious anemia affects around one in every thousand people, but is far more common in individuals over the age of sixty.

DID YOU KNOW? Pernicious anemia was a death sentence until the 1920s, when American doctors started giving their patients a diet of raw liver, which resulted in an astounding improvement. The doctors were awarded the Nobel Prize in Medicine in 1934, but vitamin B_{12} was first discovered in 1948—which made treatment far easier.

EXTRA SOURCES:

1. "Gastritt," [Gastritis] L. Aabakken, Great Norwegian Encyclopedia (online).
2. "Autoimmune Atrophic Gastritis: Current Perspectives," A. Minalyan et al., *Clinical and Experimental Gastroenterology*, 2017.
3. "Recognizing, Treating and Understanding Pernicious Anemia," L. Sinclair, *Journal of The Royal Society of Medicine*, 2008.

Autoimmune autonomic ganglionopathy

WHAT IS IT? The immune system attacks parts of the autonomic nervous system—the non-voluntary part of the nervous system, which controls central bodily functions such as body temperature, blood pressure, respiration, and digestion. Around a third of those affected seem to get better without treatment.

DID YOU KNOW? Around 60 percent of cases occur following an infection or other disease.

Autoimmune encephalitis

WHAT IS IT? Inflammation in the brain is often caused by infections, but in some cases an autoimmune reaction may be the cause. Such autoimmune reactions may occur on their own, or in connection with cancer (see *paraneoplastic syndrome*). One of the best known is anti-NMDA receptor encephalitis.

Autoimmune enteropathy

WHAT IS IT? The immune system attacks the cells that line the digestive tract, which results in uncontrollable diarrhea and problems absorbing nutrients. Most common in infants before the age of six months, but may also affect adults. The condition is life-threatening and must be treated with immunosuppressive medications and the infusion of nutrients.

DID YOU KNOW? In infants with uncontrollable (intractable) diarrhea, it seems that autoimmune enteropathy may be the cause in up to a third of cases.

EXTRA SOURCES:
1. "Autoimmune Enteropathy: A Review and Update of Clinical Management," N. M. Gentile et al., *Current Gastroenterology Reports*, 2014.
2. "Pediatric Autoimmune Enteropathy: An Entity Frequently Associated With Immunodeficiency Disorders," A. D. Singhi et al., *Modern Pathology*, 2013.

Autoimmune hemolytic anemia

WHAT IS IT? The immune system attacks the red blood cells, which results in a low blood count (anemia). Autoimmunity is the cause in around 30 percent of cases. Often occurs together with other autoimmune diseases or certain types of cancer. Symptoms may include heart palpitations, headaches, labored breathing, fatigue, dizziness, jaundice, blood in the urine, and an enlarged spleen. Removal of the spleen may be advised in certain cases. When children are affected the disease often passes, while in adults it often recurs.

DID YOU KNOW? In serious cases, the lifetime of the red blood cells is reduced from the normal 100–120 days to just a few days.

Autoimmune hepatitis

WHAT IS IT? The immune system attacks the liver, which results in inflammation. Exists in the forms type 1 and type 2. Around 80 percent of those affected have type 1; type 2 is more serious and mainly affects children and young adults. Progression of the disease varies, from few symptoms to liver failure. Patients may experience poor overall health, fatigue, nausea, stomach pain, itching, joint pain, and jaundice. In eight out of every ten people affected the disease recedes within three years, but patients often require maintenance treatment. Some require a liver transplant.

DID YOU KNOW? Without treatment, most patients die within ten years. With treatment, the mortality rate is reduced to less than 10 percent.

Autoimmune hypoparathyroidism

WHAT IS IT? Parathyroid hormone regulates the level of calcium in the body, and the glands that secrete this hormone are located just behind the thyroid gland, at the front of the throat. Hypoparathyroidism means that the individual secretes abnormally low levels of this hormone. This may result in muscle twitches and cramps, and a range of other symptoms, such as hair loss and brittle nails. The cause is generally removal of the thyroid gland, for example due to cancer. But in very rare cases the cause may be an autoimmune reaction. The condition is treated by normalizing the calcium level in the blood, and the prognosis is then good.

DID YOU KNOW? Hypoparathyroidism may result in personality changes, depression, and memory loss. In children, it may cause growth disorders and slow the child's mental development.

Autoimmune inner ear disease (AIED)

WHAT IS IT? The immune system attacks the cells of the inner ear, resulting in hearing loss on both sides. The hearing loss is sensorineural, i.e., due to a disease in or damage to the cochlea, auditory nerve, or central nervous system. Develops rapidly over weeks or months. Over half of those affected improve following treatment with corticosteroids.

DID YOU KNOW? The disease was discovered in 1979 and is the only form of sensorineural hearing loss that can be treated using medications.

Autoimmune lymphocytic hypophysitis

WHAT IS IT? Cells of the immune system infiltrate the pituitary gland, which then becomes enlarged and functions more poorly. This may result in headaches, visual disturbances, fatigue, dizziness, and nausea. Researchers believe an autoimmune reaction is involved. Some of those affected become well again without treatment; surgery is necessary in some cases. The majority of patients require lifelong treatment with hormone replacement.

DID YOU KNOW? It was originally believed that the disease only occurred in women in the period directly after birth, but more recently it has been found to affect individuals of all ages, including men.

EXTRA SOURCE: "Lymphocytic and Granulocytic Hypophysitis: A Single Centre Experience," N. Buxton et al., *British Journal of Neurosurgery*, 2001.

Autoimmune lymphoproliferative syndrome

WHAT IS IT? The body becomes unable to regulate the number of lymphocytes, a group of cells in the immune system. Overproduction of these cells results in the accumulation of lymphocytes in the lymph nodes, liver, and spleen. This often leads to autoimmune reactions and diseases, and the blood cells are most commonly affected. The disease is genetic, often starting in childhood and developing throughout the patient's life. Patients have an increased risk of cancers of the immune system.

DID YOU KNOW? In the majority of cases the patient has inherited a mutation on the FAS gene—a gene that encodes one of several proteins important to apoptosis, the normal process through which cells die. Researchers believe, however, that this mutation may also occur during the course of an individual's life, without it having to be inherited.

EXTRA SOURCE: "Autoimmune Lymphoproliferative Syndrome," J. Bleesing et al., *GenReviews*, 2017.

Autoimmune neutropenia

WHAT IS IT? The immune system starts to attack the immune system cells called neutrophils, resulting in fewer of these cells in the body. The condition most frequently affects children under the age of two, and almost all of those affected recover completely before the age of five. However, the condition may affect individuals of all ages and occur in patients suffering from other autoimmune diseases.

DID YOU KNOW? Alloimmune neutropenia occurs when autoantibodies pass from mother to child during pregnancy. The incidence is around one case per two thousand births. The condition passes within a few months.

EXTRA SOURCE: "Kronisk Nøytropeni—Inndeling og Behandling," [Chronic neutropenia—classification and treatment] H. F. Amundsen et al., *Journal of the Norwegian Medical Association*, 2003.

Autoimmune ovarian / testicular inflammation

WHAT IS IT? Inflammation that affects the ovaries or testicles is not uncommon. This is generally caused by an infection, but in rare cases it may be due to an autoimmune attack. Often occurs in connection with another autoimmune disease. For women, the symptoms are similar to early menopause because the ovaries cease to function normally. In men, the testicles may swell and become tender. In men, the disease is linked to antibodies that attack the sperm cells, and may result in sterility.

DID YOU KNOW? Researchers have found antisperm antibodies in as many as 5–12 percent of infertile men.

EXTRA SOURCE: "Diagnosis and Classification of Autoimmune Orchitis," C. A. Silve et al., *Autoimmunity Reviews*, 2014.

Autoimmune polyglandular syndrome

WHAT IS IT? Polyglandular means "several glands." Patients have a combination of several autoimmune diseases that affect the body's endocrine system, such as Addison's disease, type 1 diabetes, and thyroiditis. Treatment is the same as for when these diseases occur alone, and the prognosis is therefore good.

DID YOU KNOW? It is not uncommon to suffer from several autoimmune diseases at the same time. For example, rheumatoid arthritis patients have a greater chance of developing type 1 diabetes or thyroiditis.

EXTRA SOURCE: "Recent Insights in the Epidemiology of Autoimmune Diseases: Improved Prevalence Estimates and Understanding of Clustering of Diseases," S. G. Cooper et al., *Journal of Autoimmunity*, November 2009.

Autoimmune progesterone dermatitis

WHAT IS IT? A recurrent rash that varies in severity at different stages of the menstrual cycle. The cause is unknown, but researchers believe that an increasing level of the hormone progesterone triggers an autoimmune reaction in the skin. Removal of the ovaries may be recommended in some cases.

DID YOU KNOW? To clarify the diagnosis, a doctor may inject a small dose of progesterone under the skin, to see whether this provokes an autoimmune reaction.

Autoimmune retinopathy

WHAT IS IT? A spectrum of conditions in which the immune system attacks the proteins in the retina. Some of them are related to cancer (paraneoplastic syndrome). Patients experience rapid and pain-free deterioration of sight in both eyes, and in the worst-case scenario may go blind. As a general rule, the best that can be hoped for is to stabilize the condition.

DID YOU KNOW? When the disease is related to cancer, visual disturbances and antibodies that attack the retina may occur long before the cancer is discovered. In one famous case, the cancer was only discovered eleven years later.

EXTRA SOURCE: "Autoimmune Retinopathy: A Review," A. M. Canamary Jr. et al., *International Journal of Retina and Vitreous*, 2018.

Autoimmune stiff-person syndrome

WHAT IS IT? The immune system attacks the brain and spinal cord, which affects the neurotransmitters central to muscle function. The muscles gradually become stiffer, and this is often accompanied by spasms. Strong emotions and movements may trigger an attack, and patients may move slowly to prevent this. Some patients function normally; others experience a significant reduction in physical ability.

DID YOU KNOW? The syndrome may affect infants (stiff baby syndrome), but this variant of the condition is milder and those affected tend to grow out of it. Attacks often occur when the child is stressed or frightened.

Autoimmune uveitis

WHAT IS IT? Inflammation of the pigmented parts of the eye, including the iris. May be caused by infections, but is often due to autoimmune reactions. Symptoms may include visual disturbances, pain, sensitivity to light, and runny eyes. May occur alone or together with other autoimmune diseases. In acute cases, the patient often gets better with treatment. In cases of chronic uveitis, complications occur more often.

DID YOU KNOW? Anterior uveitis may often be the first sign of ankylosing spondylitis. Around every third patient with ankylosing spondylitis will develop anterior uveitis at some point during the course of the illness.

EXTRA SOURCES:

1. "Uveitt," [Uveitis] K. Sandvig, Great Norwegian Encyclopedia (online).
2. *Autoimmunity: From Bench to Bedside*, Juan-Manuel Anaya et al., eds., El Rosario University Press, 2013.

Celiac disease

WHAT IS IT? The immune system reacts abnormally to gluten and attacks the villi that line the small intestine, which are central in the absorption of nutrients. This results in inflammation in the digestive system. Affects around 1 percent of the population in the West, and is one of the most common autoimmune diseases. Usual symptoms include stomach pain, loose stools, weight loss, and fatigue. Celiac disease is more genetic than many other autoimmune diseases. Of the individuals who have a parent with celiac disease, around 10 percent will also develop the disease. Almost all sufferers become healthy when following a gluten-free diet.

DID YOU KNOW? Finland and Ireland have the highest incidence of celiac disease in the world. Inhabitants of Southeast Asia and sub-Saharan Africa rarely develop celiac disease.

Chronic inflammatory demyelinating polyneuropathy (CIDP)

WHAT IS IT? The immune system attacks the insulation (myelin) around the peripheral nerves, which results in weakness, paralysis, numbness, and pain. Some patients become progressively worse; others experience periods in which their symptoms worsen and improve. Around half of those affected improve so much over the course of a year that they no longer require treatment. After a few years, almost nine out of every ten patients have no, or only very little, reduction in function.

DID YOU KNOW? CIDP is a chronic form of Guillain-Barré syndrome.

Chronic urticaria

WHAT IS IT? Urticaria is more commonly known as hives, an itchy rash consisting of raised bumps and welts of various sizes. The mast cells release histamine, which causes the rash. The condition is often an allergic reaction or triggered by an infection. If it lasts for over six weeks, it is termed chronic urticaria, and researchers believe it to be due to an autoimmune attack on the mast cells. In most cases the condition disappears after a couple of years. In Norway, hives affects one in every five people at some point during their lifetime, but the chronic variant affects a much smaller percentage.

DID YOU KNOW? In Norwegian, hives is commonly known as *elveblest,* or "elf-blown," because it was once believed that elves were responsible for blowing the disease onto humans.

EXTRA SOURCE: "Urtikaria," [Urticaria] D. S. Holsen and T. Langeland, Great Norwegian Encyclopedia (online).

Cogan's syndrome

WHAT IS IT? Attacks the eyes and the inner ear. Symptoms may include painful or red eyes, visual and auditory deterioration, sensitivity to light, dizziness, nausea, and tinnitus. Patients also often have vasculitis, inflammation of the blood vessels. The cause is unclear, but researchers believe autoimmunity plays a central role. May result in permanent damage to the patient's hearing or sight.

DID YOU KNOW? Researchers suspect autoantibodies of attacking something in the eyes and inner ear. In a study from 2002, researchers transferred this type of autoantibody to mice, which resulted in the mice developing the symptoms of Cogan's syndrome.

EXTRA SOURCES:
1. "Autoantibodies to Inner Ear and Endothelial Antigens in Cogan's Syndrome," C. Lunardi et al., *Lancet*, 2002.
2. "Cogan's Syndrome: An Autoimmune Inner Ear Disease," A. Greco et al., *Autoimmunity Reviews*, 2013.

Complex regional pain syndrome (CRPS)

WHAT IS IT? A pain condition that affects a limited area, most often an arm or a leg. Previously known as reflex sympathetic dystrophy. Often triggered by an injury in the area in question, such as a broken bone or an operation. Symptoms include intense, burning pain, and the area may swell; the skin may change color and become hypersensitive. The cause is unknown, and autoimmunity is just one of many theories; researchers have found autoantibodies against parts of the sympathetic nervous system. Most of those affected experience improvement within one to two years.

DID YOU KNOW? One of the largest studies on CRPS showed that it affects the arms more often than the legs, and that broken bones were the most common triggering factor (in 44 percent of cases).

EXTRA SOURCE: "Clinical Features and Pathophysiology of Complex Regional Pain Syndrome—Current State of the Art," J. Marinus et al., *Lancet Neurology*, 2011.

Crohn's disease

WHAT IS IT? Chronic inflammation of the digestive tract. Along with ulcerative colitis, comes under the umbrella term inflammatory bowel disease (IBD). Sufferers experience periods with few or no symptoms, and periods in which the disease flares up. With treatment the prognosis is often good. When children are affected, this may result in delayed growth and development. Complications, such as narrowing of the bowel, may make it necessary to operate. Crohn's disease is more common in northern regions, and less common in Asia and South America.

DID YOU KNOW? Crohn's may affect any part of the digestive system, from the mouth to the anus. The area where the small intestine transitions into the large intestine is most often affected.

Dermatitis herpetiformis

WHAT IS IT? The immune system attacks the skin, resulting in an itchy, spotty rash characterized by blisters filled with a watery fluid. Closely linked to celiac disease; 15–20 percent of individuals with celiac disease develop dermatitis herpetiformis. When following a gluten-free diet, patients generally experience few problems.

DID YOU KNOW? Patients often have no symptoms of gastrointestinal disease, but examinations via gastroscopy show that most have abnormal changes in the small intestine.

Diabetes, type 1

WHAT IS IT? The immune system attacks the cells of the pancreas that create insulin, which results in too little insulin being produced. Insulin is necessary for the absorption of sugar and the conversion of energy. Patients experience a period of increased thirst, frequent urination, poor overall health, and weight loss, which is then followed by an acute attack with high blood sugar. Without treatment, the patient will fall into a coma and die. Treatment with insulin and effective control of the insulin level enables patients to live a normal life. The disease often arises in childhood and young adulthood, with around half of all new cases affecting individuals over the age of twenty. There is significant geographical variation in the number of individuals affected. A Finnish child has a risk of developing type 1 diabetes that is forty times greater than that of a Japanese child.

DID YOU KNOW? Over 90 percent of people suffering from diabetes have type 2 of the disease. Type 2 diabetes is not an autoimmune disease but is linked to lifestyle factors and obesity. Across the world, over four hundred million people live with type 1 or 2 diabetes, and around 12 percent of the world's health budgets are spent on these diseases.

Encephalitis lethargica (sleeping sickness)

WHAT IS IT? In 1917, the world was hit by a mysterious epidemic that lasted for over a decade. Patients developed inflammation in the brain, and the condition was termed sleeping sickness because many of those affected ended up not being able to move or speak. Around one million people died. The cause is a mystery, and only isolated cases have since been observed. In 2004, researchers found autoantibodies that target the basal ganglia in the brain, and suggested that autoimmunity may be behind the condition. Others believe a virus damaged the brain, because the epidemic occurred at the same time as the 1918 flu pandemic.

DID YOU KNOW? In the 1960s, the medication L-Dopa was discovered as a treatment for Parkinson's disease. At that time, there were sleeping sickness patients who had been in an apathetic state for forty years. When these patients were given L-Dopa, many of them miraculously came to life, but when the medicine stopped working many returned to their helpless state. The story is described in the book *Awakenings* by doctor Oliver Sacks.

EXTRA SOURCES:
1. "Encephalitis Lethargica Syndrome: 20 New Cases and Evidence of Basal Ganglia Autoimmunity," R. C. Dale et al., *Brain*, 2004.
2. "Encephalitis Lethargica Information Page," National Institute of Neurological Disorders and Stroke, ninds.nih.gov/Disorders/All-Disorders/Encephalitis-Lethargica-Information-Page.

Eosinophilic fasciitis

WHAT IS IT? An extremely rare condition, also known as Shulman's syndrome, in which the connective tissue beneath the skin becomes inflamed, thickening and tightening. This results in swelling, and muscle and joint pain may also occur. Specific immune system cells (eosinophils) accumulate in the affected areas. The cause is unclear, but some believe the disease to be a variant of scleroderma. Most individuals affected improve with treatment.

DID YOU KNOW? It is believed that in some cases the disease is triggered by extreme physical activity.

Epidermolysis bullosa acquisita

WHAT IS IT? The immune system attacks the skin and mucous membranes, causing blisters. Often occurs after minor injuries to exposed areas such as the hands, feet, knees, elbows, and buttocks. Appears to be caused by antibodies attacking a protein in the connective tissue that anchors the skin. The disease fluctuates through periods in which the symptoms improve and worsen. Most live well with the disease.

DID YOU KNOW? Patients are advised to avoid sports that involve body contact.

Felty's syndrome

WHAT IS IT? Affects patients with rheumatoid arthritis (RA) who also have an enlarged spleen and a low neutrophil count (neutropenia). The cause is unknown, but autoimmunity is thought to be behind the disease. Some contract life-threatening infections as a result of a weakened immune system, and it may become necessary to remove the spleen.

DID YOU KNOW? One to three percent of patients with rheumatoid arthritis also develop Felty's syndrome.

Glomerulonephritis (inflammation of the kidneys)

WHAT IS IT? An umbrella term for a number of inflammatory diseases that affect the small filters (glomeruli) in the kidneys. Some of these diseases are thought to be an autoimmune reaction in which the group A *Streptococcus* bacteria seem to trigger the attack. Often few symptoms, and so generally discovered by chance from a urine sample. Sometimes patients experience rapid onset of symptoms, such as swelling in the face, fatigue, blood in the urine, headache, and nausea. May result in high blood pressure, decreased urine production, and kidney failure. Many of those affected make a full recovery, but some become seriously ill and require dialysis. In around 25 percent of patients with kidney failure, glomerulonephritis is the cause. A kidney transplant may be necessary.

DID YOU KNOW? Western countries have experienced a significant decrease in kidney inflammation due to streptococci, probably due to the use of antibiotics. In less-developed countries the condition is still fairly common.

RELATED CONDITION: Goodpasture syndrome, in which a specific type of autoantibody (anti-GBM) attacks both the kidneys and lungs. Results in glomerulonephritis and bleeding in the lungs and is fatal without treatment. With aggressive treatment, over 80 percent of patients live with the disease for over five years.

Graves' disease

WHAT IS IT? The immune system produces antibodies similar to thyroid stimulating hormone (TSH). This causes the thyroid gland to increase the metabolism, and is the most common cause of an overactive thyroid (hyperthyroidism). Affects around 0.5 percent of men and 3 percent of women at some point during their life. Symptoms may include heart palpitations, weight loss, sweating, fatigue, diarrhea, shaking, difficulty sleeping, and irritability. Is treated using medications that inhibit production of the thyroid hormones, or with radiation or surgery. Some of those affected become completely symptom-free, while others develop serious complications. Radiation and surgery destroy the thyroid gland, and the patient must then receive replacement hormones for life.

DID YOU KNOW? More than one in every ten patients develops Graves' eye disease, which causes protruding, bulging eyes.

EXTRA SOURCE: "Management of Graves' Disease: A Review," H. B. Burch et al., *JAMA*, 2015.

Guillain-Barré syndrome

WHAT IS IT? The immune system destroys the insulation (myelin) that surrounds the nerves of the peripheral nervous system. Seems to be triggered by an infection, often in the airways or gut. Affects the lower part of the body first, with tingling, burning pains, and weakness in the muscles, which then spreads upward. May affect the breathing muscles, and one in three patients require a respirator. In most patients, the spread of the disease stops after a month. Around 80 percent of those affected make a full recovery, but this often takes months. Some suffer long-term neurological damage; a few experience a serious reduction in physical ability.

DID YOU KNOW? The infection that most often triggers Guillain-Barré syndrome is from the *Campylobacter* bacteria, a common cause of food poisoning.

SUBTYPES: The description above applies to the most common form of the disease: acute inflammatory demyelinating polyneuropathy. According to the Norwegian Online Medical Handbook, there are also eleven other subdiagnoses.

Hashimoto's thyroiditis

WHAT IS IT? The immune system attacks the thyroid gland. Patients first experience a high metabolism, which then dips to a low metabolism. Symptoms may include fatigue, constipation, weight gain, increased sensitivity to cold, joint and muscle pain, decreased sweat production, depression, high blood pressure, and hair loss. The thyroid gland often swells (goiter). With hormone replacement therapy, most patients live normal lives.

DID YOU KNOW? Hashimoto's syndrome is the most common disease that causes low metabolism, but worldwide it is iodine deficiency that most often causes low metabolism.

Idiopathic thrombocytopenic purpura (ITP)

WHAT IS IT? The immune system attacks the platelets in the blood—this is the most common cause of a low platelet count. Results in bleeding in the skin, similar to bruises. The condition is often temporary in children (in over 80 percent of cases), but chronic in adults. In most cases a benign disease, but significant bleeding can be serious, especially in the head. Around 1 percent of affected children and 5 percent of affected adults die of serious bleeding.

DID YOU KNOW? It may be necessary to remove the spleen, since this suppresses the immune system. Patients must then be followed up with extra vaccines and more aggressive use of antibiotics in the case of infections.

IgG4-related diseases

WHAT IS IT? A range of conditions that may affect almost any of the body's organs. Results in inflammation and fibrosis (scarring). The attacked organs swell in a way that is reminiscent of cancer. Those affected have greater than normal numbers of a group of antibodies known as IgG4. These conditions were previously regarded as unrelated diagnoses, and have only been gathered under the umbrella term IgG4-related diseases in recent years. Most patients get better, but recurrence is common.

DID YOU KNOW? The prototype IgG4-related disease is autoimmune pancreatitis, which attacks the pancreas and other organs. It was in patients with this condition that researchers first discovered high levels of IgG4, in 2001.

EXTRA SOURCES:

1. "IgG4-Relatert Sykdom," [IgG4-related diseases] J. Vikse et al., *Journal of the Norwegian Medical Association*, 2017.
2. "High Serum IgG4 Concentrations in Patients With Sclerosing Pancreatitis," H. Hamano et al., *New England Journal of Medicine*, 2001.

Interstitial cystitis

WHAT IS IT? Also known as painful bladder syndrome. Symptoms include pelvic pain, frequent urination, and the feeling of constantly needing to pee. Fluctuates through periods in which symptoms worsen and improve. The cause is unknown, and the diagnosis much discussed. A study estimated that 2–6 percent of American women have the symptoms of the disease, but less than 10 percent of these had been diagnosed. Autoimmunity is just one of many theories, but autoantibodies have been found in those affected, and the condition seems to be linked to several autoimmune diseases.

DID YOU KNOW? Patients are more likely to have experienced cystitis, gynecological operations, and bladder problems during childhood.

EXTRA SOURCE: "Sub-Noxious Intravesical Lipopolysaccharide Triggers Bladder Inflammation and Symptom Onset in a Transgenic Autoimmune Cystitis Model: A MAPP Network Animal Study," P. Kogan et al., *Scientific Reports*, 2018.

IPEX syndrome

WHAT IS IT? IPEX stands for "immune dysregulation, polyendocrinopathy, enteropathy, X-linked." Affects only boys and starts before the age of six months. Caused by a mutation on the FOXP3 gene, which destroys the function of the regulating T cells. The result is a number of autoimmune attacks. Common symptoms include severe diarrhea, diabetes, rashes, and thyroiditis. Without treatment, most of those affected die within two years.

DID YOU KNOW? According to an article from 2011, the medical literature describes fewer than 150 individuals with IPEX syndrome.

EXTRA SOURCE: "IPEX Syndrome," M. C. Hannibal et al., *Gene Reviews*, 2011.

Isaacs' syndrome

WHAT IS IT? A neuromuscular disease that results in hyperactive peripheral nerves. May cause twitching and spasms in the muscles, muscle stiffness that gradually worsens over time, and increased sweating. The cause is unknown, but researchers believe autoimmunity to play a central role in a number of cases. Often occurs with certain cancers or other autoimmune diseases. The prognosis varies depending on the patient's additional diagnoses.

DID YOU KNOW? The symptoms, such as contracting and twitching muscles and sweating, continue even when the patient is sleeping or under general anesthetic.

Juvenile idiopathic arthritis

WHAT IS IT? The immune system attacks the joints in children. This results in inflammation, causing swelling, pain, and stiffness in the joints. The symptoms come and go, and depend on the type of juvenile arthritis. The systemic form may attack the internal organs, resulting in poor overall general health and a high fever, but this is only responsible for less than 5 percent of cases. Many children affected by the disease become completely free of it, while some may experience aftereffects as adults. This is the most common rheumatic disease in children.

DID YOU KNOW? A study showed that children who have received antibiotics are more at risk of developing juvenile idiopathic arthritis. Researchers have speculated on whether this is because antibiotics change the body's internal bacterial flora, but additional studies have not confirmed this finding.

STILL'S DISEASE: Juvenile idiopathic arthritis was previously called Still's disease. Adults may develop a disease reminiscent of juvenile idiopathic arthritis, which is then called adult-onset Still's disease.

Lambert–Eaton myasthenic syndrome

WHAT IS IT? The immune system attacks the calcium channels at the transitional points between the nerves and muscles, and in the autonomic nervous system. This inhibits acetylcholine, an important neurotransmitter within the nervous system. Patients develop muscle weakness and autonomic symptoms such as dryness of the mouth and impotence. Around half of those who develop the syndrome are affected in connection with some form of cancer.

DID YOU KNOW? Small cell lung cancer is the most common form of cancer associated with the syndrome. Patients who develop Lambert–Eaton myasthenic syndrome have a better cancer prognosis than those who don't develop the syndrome, possibly because it enables earlier detection of the cancer.

Lichen planus

WHAT IS IT? The immune system attacks the cells of the skin and mucous membranes, which leads to inflammation and an itchy rash. May affect the skin, hair, nails, and mucous membranes of the mouth or genitals. Seems to be linked to the hepatitis C infection, in addition to several other autoimmune diseases. Often goes away by itself within one to two years.

DID YOU KNOW? Certain types of drugs, such as antimalarials and blood pressure medications, seem to trigger lichen planus in some individuals.

Lichen sclerosus

WHAT IS IT? An inflammatory disease that primarily affects the genitals and area around the anus in women, but may also affect men. Studies have shown that it affects one in every thousand girls before puberty, and 3 percent of elderly women in nursing homes. Causes itching and pain. The skin takes on the appearance of cigarette paper, i.e., thin, white, and wrinkled. The cause is unknown, but several researchers believe autoimmunity plays a role in some cases. Often goes away by itself.

DID YOU KNOW? The condition occurs most frequently in women after menopause and in girls before puberty. The use of the contraceptive pill just before menopause increases the risk of developing the condition, which indicates that hormones play an important role.

Ménière's disease

WHAT IS IT? Affects the inner ear and leads to dizzy spells, hearing loss, tinnitus, and pressure in the ear. Often starts in one ear but may later affect both. The cause is unknown, but the accumulation of fluid is found in parts of the inner ear. Some researchers believe autoimmunity to be the cause in a number of cases. For most patients, the disease eases off or stabilizes after a few years. Many have long-term problems with poor balance and hearing.

DID YOU KNOW? Prosper Ménière described the disease in 1861. At the time, the condition was known as "glaucoma of the ear." Glaucoma is an eye disease, in which the pressure inside the eye is too high.

EXTRA SOURCES:

1. "Ménière's Disease Might Be an Autoimmune Condition?" A.Greco et al., *Autoimmunity Reviews*, 2012.

2. "Autoimmunity as a Candidate for the Etiopathogenesis of Meniere's Disease: Detection of Autoimmune Reactions and Diagnostic Biomarker Candidate," S. H. Kim et al., *PLoS One*, 2014.

Mixed connective tissue disease (MCTD)

WHAT IS IT? An inflammatory disease of the connective tissue, which is thought to be due to an autoimmune reaction. Patients develop fibrosis, where the tissue becomes hard and stiff. Common symptoms include joint pain, fatigue, swollen hands, Raynaud's phenomenon, and lung problems. Most people live well with the disease, but a few of those affected develop serious complications in the heart and lungs.

DID YOU KNOW? It can take a long time to be properly diagnosed because the disease changes over time. One Norwegian study showed an average of 3.6 years passed between the appearance of the first symptoms and diagnosis of the disease.

Morvan's syndrome

WHAT IS IT? The immune system attacks both the peripheral and central nervous system. Most of those affected have antibodies against a protein that is important for communication in parts of the nervous system. The nervous system becomes hyperactive. May result in convulsions and twitching muscles, fluctuations in blood pressure, persistent insomnia, hallucinations, confusion, pain, and weight loss. Treatment is effective, but a number of those affected experience recurrences.

DID YOU KNOW? Patients often experience twitching of the muscles that can look like a nest of vipers beneath the skin.

EXTRA SOURCES:

1. "Morvan Just a Syndrome ...!" E. R. Somerville et al., *Lancet*, 2017.

2. "From VGKC to LGI1 and Caspr 2 Encephalitis: The Evolution of a Disease Entity Over Time," A. van Sonderen et al., *Autoimmunity Reviews*, 2016.

Multiple sclerosis (MS)

WHAT IS IT? The immune system attacks the insulation (myelin) around the nerves, which results in inflammation in the central nervous system. The incidence of MS increases the farther you get from the equator. In Europe and North America, one to two inhabitants in every thousand have MS. Symptoms include visual disturbances, paralysis, fatigue, poor body control, problems urinating, and much more. Patients experience episodic attacks. A few of those affected develop a progressive form of the disease, in which their condition gradually worsens. The aim of treatment is to prevent new attacks.

DID YOU KNOW? MS may affect children as young as two years old, but this is extremely rare.

Myasthenia gravis

WHAT IS IT? The immune system attacks the area where the nervous system transfers signals to the muscles. The main symptom is muscle weakness that gets worse with activity and improves after rest. The eyes are often affected first, with double vision and droopy eyelids. The disease spreads, and in some cases can affect all the muscles under voluntary control. With treatment, most live a normal life. In younger patients it is possible to remove the thymus, which cures some individuals, but such operations involve certain risks.

DID YOU KNOW? Previously, 30–40 percent of patients died. With current treatment, the mortality rate has been reduced to 3–4 percent.

Myocarditis

WHAT IS IT? Inflammation of the heart muscle. May be caused by infections or poisonous substances, but is most often an auto-immune reaction. Some experience no or only mild symptoms; others experience acute heart failure and may die. The condition generally goes away, but some of those affected develop chronic inflammation and gradually develop the symptoms of heart failure. Treatment is often unnecessary, but patients must be monitored. A pacemaker or heart transplant is recommended in a few cases.

DID YOU KNOW? Myocarditis is one of the most common causes of sudden death in otherwise healthy young people.

Myositis

WHAT IS IT? The immune system attacks the tissue of the muscles, such as the blood vessels, connective tissue, and muscle cells. It is divided into three groups: polymyositis, dermatomyositis, and inclusion body myositis. Symptoms include muscle weakness and pain, particularly in the shoulders and hips. Most of those affected by polymyositis and dermatomyositis get better; around one in every three patients makes a full recovery. In the case of inclusion body myositis, treatment is less effective. Without treatment, the result is often significant physical impairment, and the condition may be life-threatening.

DID YOU KNOW? Some studies indicate that strong UV radiation increases the risk of myositis.

Neuromyelitis optica

WHAT IS IT? The immune system attacks the insulation (myelin) around the nerves in the spinal cord and eyes. Symptoms may include paralysis, pain, numbness and tingling in the spine, arms and legs, vision loss, and problems urinating. Was once thought to be a form of multiple sclerosis, but in 2004 researchers discovered an autoantibody against a protein associated with the blood-brain barrier. Patients often develop permanent muscle failure, paralysis, and sight loss within five years. For 25–50 percent of those affected, the disease is ultimately fatal.

DID YOU KNOW? The disease was previously called Devic's disease after Eugène Devic, who described sixteen patients with the disease in 1894. Even back then, some doctors believed the disease to be different from MS, but it would be over a hundred years before researchers finally determined that it was in fact a separate disease.

EXTRA SOURCE: "Neuromyelitis Optica," S. Kvistad et al., *Journal of the Norwegian Medical Association*, 2013.

Optic neuritis (inflammation of the optic nerve)

WHAT IS IT? The immune system attacks the insulation around the optic nerve, which transmits information from the retina to the brain. Often occurs in connection with multiple sclerosis or neuromyelitis optica, but may also occur alone. Vision loss occurs over the course of hours or days, and the eye often becomes painful and tender, often only on one side. The condition often improves without treatment. Normal vision returns in more than nine in ten patients.

DID YOU KNOW? Inflammation of the optic nerve may be the first sign of MS. Up to 75 percent of affected female patients and 35 percent of male patients are later diagnosed with MS.

Palindromic rheumatism

WHAT IS IT? Periodic inflammation in one or more joints, lasting from a few hours to several days. The fingers, wrists, and knees are most commonly affected. Patients are symptom-free between attacks, and months may pass between one attack and the next. The cause is unknown, but autoimmunity is thought to play a role, especially as the disease is closely related to rheumatoid arthritis (RA). Around a third of those affected will later develop RA.

DID YOU KNOW? A palindrome is a word that reads the same forward and backward, such as "radar" or "level." The disease was given its name because the attacks build up toward a peak before gradually disappearing again.

EXTRA SOURCE: *Palindromic Rheumatism*, Arthritis Research UK, versusarthritis.org/media/1338/palindromic-rheumatism-information-booklet.pdf.

PANDAS

WHAT IS IT? Stands for "pediatric autoimmune neuropsychiatric disorders associated with streptococcal infections," a hypothesis that obsessive-compulsive disorder or tics occur acutely in children after a streptococcal infection. Affects children between the ages of three and twelve years. Anxiety attacks, problems sleeping, attention deficit hyperactivity disorder symptoms, joint pain, and mood swings may last for weeks or months. The cause is unclear, but some researchers believe the immune system attacks areas of the brain because they are similar to *Streptococcus* bacteria. This diagnosis was established in 1998 and is contentious because the connection to *Streptococcus* is not proven.

DID YOU KNOW? American researchers believe that they have created a PANDAS-like disease in mice. They transferred a specific type of antibody from mice with PANDAS to healthy mice, which resulted in behavioral changes in the healthy mice.

EXTRA SOURCE: "Passive Transfer of Streptococcus-Induced Antibodies Reproduces Behavioral Disturbances in a Mouse Model of Pediatric Autoimmune Neuropsychiatric Disorders Associated With Streptococcal Infection," K. Yaddanapudi et al., *Molecular Psychiatry*, 2010.

Paraneoplastic syndrome

WHAT IS IT? A group of conditions that affects less than 1 percent of cancer patients. The immune system attacks the nervous system, which can result in a range of symptoms. Several of the paraneoplastic syndromes result from the cells of the immune system confusing the nervous tissue with the cancer cells they are trying to destroy. Most patients develop neurological symptoms before the cancer is discovered and diagnosed. The prognosis varies, from full recovery to death.

DID YOU KNOW? Several autoimmune diseases may be a paraneoplastic syndrome in some cases, but not in others. This means that one patient may develop the disease as a result of a malignant tumor, while others may develop the same disease without any such tumor being present.

EXTRA SOURCE: "Paraneoplastiske Nevrologiske Syndromer," [Paraneoplastic neurological syndromes] A. Storstein et al., *Journal of the Norwegian Medical Association*, 2009.

Parry–Romberg syndrome

WHAT IS IT? Affects the skin and soft tissues of the face, generally only on the left side. The tissue slowly shrinks (atrophies), causing the face to become deformed. May also affect the arms and legs. Starts mostly in childhood, around the age of ten. Many researchers believe it to be a form of scleroderma, and caused by an autoimmune attack. Most of those affected become gradually worse over the course of two to twenty years, before the condition stabilizes.

DID YOU KNOW? In serious cases the syndrome results in extreme deformation of the face, and cosmetic surgery then becomes necessary.

Parsonage-Turner syndrome

WHAT IS IT? Also known as brachial plexopathy or neuralgic amyotrophy. The characteristic symptoms are acute and intense pain in the shoulder and chest on one side of the body. Paralysis occurs within days. Researchers believe autoimmunity plays a central role. Ninety percent of patients recover normal function within three years.

DID YOU KNOW? Up to one in every four patients with this condition is repeatedly affected.

Pemphigoid

WHAT IS IT? The immune system attacks the structures of the skin, resulting in fluid-filled blisters and itching. Affects the skin more deeply than the related pemphigus (see below). Often occurs on skin that is extensively bent and stretched, such as elbows and kneecaps. Around a third of those affected are also attacked in the mucous membranes of the mouth, genitals, and anus. The disease is often prolonged, but may also disappear after a few years.

DID YOU KNOW? Some studies indicate that insect bites, such as those of sandflies and bedbugs, may trigger the disease.

Pemphigus

WHAT IS IT? The immune system attacks the cells of the skin and mucous membranes, affecting the proteins that hold the cells together. Causes large blisters. Two main types: pemphigus vulgaris (most common), and pemphigus foliaceus. In the latter, only the skin is affected, but in the former the blisters often first appear in the mouth. Aggressive treatment is important, and over half of those affected are symptom-free after five years. Without treatment the disease is fatal.

DID YOU KNOW? In a study from an isolated area of Brazil, an entire 2.6 percent of the Indigenous population was affected by pemphigus foliaceus.

Polymyalgia rheumatica (PMR)

WHAT IS IT? An inflammatory condition that mainly affects elderly individuals. Common symptoms include pain in the muscles and joints of the shoulders and hips, morning stiffness, fever, fatigue, and headache. The cause is unknown, but autoimmunity is thought to play a role. Corticosteroids often provide dramatic improvement in just a few hours, and the prognosis is excellent. Around every fourth patient experiences a recurrence.

DID YOU KNOW? The disease is far more common in Northern Europe than farther south. Scandinavia is among the areas of the world with the highest incidence.

Post-cardiac injury syndrome

WHAT IS IT? Inflammation affects the sac surrounding the heart (pericardium). Generally triggered by an injury in the area, often heart surgery. The injury seems to release substances that cause the immune system to attack the heart tissue. Most cases go away within a few weeks, and the condition rarely lasts over six months.

DID YOU KNOW? Cardiac tamponade is an extremely uncommon but serious complication. The sac around the heart fills with fluid, which inhibits the heart's function and may result in a heart attack.

Primary biliary cholangitis (primary biliary cirrhosis)

WHAT IS IT? The immune system attacks the small bile ducts of the liver, destroying them. The body becomes unable to transport bile to the gut, and so it accumulates. The disease often starts with tiredness and itching, followed by greasy stools, bloody vomit, and jaundice. Becomes gradually worse over the years. A liver transplant was previously necessary, but since the development of bile acid treatment most patients now no longer require this. The course of the disease varies, but with early treatment many live normal lives. Patients do, however, have an increased risk of dying earlier than normal.

DID YOU KNOW? Individuals who have a parent or sibling with the disease have a risk of developing the disease that is one thousand times greater than that of others. However, since the disease is extremely rare, the chance is still low. Researchers wonder whether this increased risk is due to the inheritance of a poorly regulated immune system.

Primary sclerosing cholangitis

WHAT IS IT? Inflammation occurs in the bile ducts, which transfer bile from the liver to the gut. The ducts eventually become blocked. Up to 90 percent of those affected also have ulcerative colitis. The cause is unknown, but autoimmunity is thought to play a central role. At first, there are often few symptoms. Tiredness, itching, pain in the upper part of the stomach, and jaundice are then common. There are few good treatment alternatives, and the liver finally fails. Liver transplantation is advised for patients under sixty-five. On average, patients live for twelve years after having been diagnosed.

DID YOU KNOW? Smokers seem to have less risk of developing the disease.

Psoriasis

WHAT IS IT? The immune system attacks the skin, resulting in chronic inflammation and a red, scaly rash that may also itch. Two to three percent of the population has psoriasis. Typically affects the elbows, knees, and back, but may appear anywhere on the body. There is significant variation in how severely individuals are affected, and the disease may flare up throughout the patient's life. Stress, infections, alcohol, and medicines may trigger outbreaks. If both parents have psoriasis, there is around a 60 percent chance that the child will also develop the condition.

DID YOU KNOW? In a study of 26,000 South American Indigenous people, researchers found not a single case of psoriasis.

Psoriatic arthritis

WHAT IS IT? A form of arthritis that affects 5 to 30 percent of people with psoriasis. Mostly affects the hands and feet, but also affects the back and pelvis in around one third of those affected. The disease is generally mild, with limited symptoms. Some develop a more aggressive variant that results in physical impairment. Treated with immunosuppressive medicines or surgery.

DID YOU KNOW? May also affect children. Juvenile psoriatic arthritis most often occurs around the age of five in girls, while boys are often affected some years later.

Pyoderma gangrenosum

WHAT IS IT? Causes sores on the skin, and may also affect the internal organs. Often appears as deep sores, which are usually violet or blue in color. May be reminiscent of midge bites or pimples, which then eventually merge into a large sore. Half of those affected also have another disease, such as rheumatoid arthritis or inflammatory bowel disease. The cause is unknown, but it is suspected that autoimmune reactions are involved. The prognosis is good with rapid treatment, but recurrences are common, and scarring often occurs.

DID YOU KNOW? Researchers believe the disease is linked to the cells of the immune system called neutrophils. Some error in the system possibly lures these cells to the site of the damage (a process called chemotaxis—cells moving in response to a stimulus).

Raynaud's phenomenon

WHAT IS IT? The blood vessels contract, reducing the blood supply to the fingers and toes. An extremely common condition, which affects up to 5 percent of the population. Stress and cold may trigger attacks. The color of the skin often changes from pale (lack of blood) to blue (too little oxygen) to red (the blood suddenly returning). May occur as a secondary condition in patients with autoimmune diseases, but most often occurs alone (primary variant). The cause is unknown, but researchers suspect autoimmunity.

DID YOU KNOW? Individuals with Raynaud's phenomenon seem to have a risk of migraine four times greater than that of non-sufferers.

EXTRA SOURCES:

1. "Prevalence, Risk Factors and Associations of Primary Raynaud's Phenomenon: Systematic Review and Meta-Analysis of Observational Studies," R. Garner et al., BMJ *Open*, 2015.

2. "An Autoimmune Basis for Raynaud's Phenomenon: Murine Model and Human Disease," D. P. Ascherman et al., *Arthritis & Rheumatology*, 2018.

Reactive arthritis

WHAT IS IT? The immune system attacks the joints and tendons. Various bacterial infections trigger the disease, including intestinal bacteria such as *Salmonella* and *Shigella*, as well as the bacteria that cause sexually transmitted infections such as chlamydia and gonorrhea. Around 80 percent of those affected have the HLA-B27 gene. In most patients, the condition goes away within a few months, but around 15 percent develop chronic symptoms.

DID YOU KNOW? Hans Reiter first described the disease in 1916, and it was therefore called Reiter's syndrome. Reiter was later convicted of war crimes, having performed medical experiments at Buchenwald concentration camp. Consequently, the term Reiter's syndrome is now not widely used.

Relapsing polychondritis

WHAT IS IT? Chondritis is inflammation of the cartilage. It often affects the ears, nose, and airways. Joint pain is common. The cause is unknown, but an autoimmune reaction probably plays a central role. Every third patient also has another autoimmune disease. Chondritis appears in periodic attacks and generally gets worse over time. It may result in vision and hearing loss, balance problems, and cardiovascular disease. Can be life-threatening, but two of every three patients live for at least five years after diagnosis.

DID YOU KNOW? Up to half of the deaths associated with the disease are a result of complications relating to the airways.

Rheumatic fever

WHAT IS IT? An inflammatory disease that may affect the joints, heart, blood vessels, central nervous system, and skin. Occurs following a streptococcal infection, where the immune system confuses healthy tissue with the *Streptococcus*. Usually goes away within a couple of weeks with treatment. Often affects the valves of the heart—patients develop rheumatic heart disease, which may be life-threatening. Extremely rare in developed countries due to good hygiene and the use of antibiotics, but the disease still causes around 300,000 deaths per year in developing countries.

DID YOU KNOW? Worldwide, around 470,000 new cases of the disease are diagnosed each year. Around 60 percent of those affected develop rheumatic heart disease; fifteen million people live with such heart problems.

Rheumatoid arthritis

WHAT IS IT? The immune system attacks the joints and causes inflammation. Over time, this may spread to the internal organs. Rheumatoid arthritis is one of the most common autoimmune diseases, affecting 0.5–1 percent of the population. Generally starts in the small joints of the hands and feet and affects both sides of the body. In 10–15 percent of those affected, the disease starts suddenly, with symptoms presenting in several joints. Patients experience periods of improvement and relapse. Some live fairly normal lives, while others experience severe functional impairment. Research from the United States shows that almost 40 percent of patients are physically disabled ten years after having received a diagnosis.

DID YOU KNOW? Around 70 percent of patients have the auto-antibody rheumatoid factor (RF) in their blood. Norwegian Erik Waaler discovered RF by chance in 1937, when he ran a syphilis test on a patient who was also suffering from rheumatoid arthritis.

Sarcoidosis

WHAT IS IT? An inflammatory disease that primarily affects the lungs, with the appearance of lumps known as granulomas. The nervous system and heart may also be affected. The cause is unknown, but autoimmunity is thought to play a role. In most cases the condition goes away by itself, but in the worst-case scenario the disease may be fatal. Scandinavia is the area of the world with the greatest number of new cases of the disease in relation to the population.

DID YOU KNOW? Those who helped to clear away the rubble at the site of the World Trade Center following the terrorist attacks on September 11, 2001, may have developed sarcoidosis at an increased rate. Researchers have long suspected that there is more risk of developing the disease among certain occupational groups, such as construction workers, miners, and farmers.

Scleritis

WHAT IS IT? The sclera is the white outer coating of the eye. Scleritis is an autoimmune attack on the sclera, which results in inflammation. May affect one or both eyes. Often occurs in connection with another autoimmune disease, such as rheumatoid arthritis or vasculitis. Symptoms include painful, red eyes. The prognosis varies, from a condition that will clear up by itself to vision loss.

DID YOU KNOW? Two-thirds of patients require treatment using high doses of corticosteroids.

RELATED CONDITION: Episcleritis, or inflammation of the episclera, which is the clear layer on top of the white part of the eye. Far more common than scleritis, and often goes away by itself within a couple of weeks. The cause is unknown, but an autoimmune reaction is also suspected here.

Sjögren's syndrome

WHAT IS IT? The immune system attacks the body's glands, particularly the tear and salivary glands, which results in inflammation. Affects 0.5–1.5 percent of the population, and nine out of ten of those affected are women. Patients experience symptoms that include dry eyes and a dry mouth. Dryness in the mouth can lead to dental problems, and so dentists are often first to identify the disease. Most patients are only mildly affected.

DID YOU KNOW? The condition is closely related to several auto-immune diseases, such as rheumatoid arthritis and systemic lupus erythematosus.

Susac's syndrome

WHAT IS IT? Affects the small blood vessels in the brain, the eyes, and the inner ear. The cause is unknown, but an autoimmune reaction is thought to be involved. Common symptoms include vision and hearing loss, headache, problems walking normally, memory loss, and confusion. Most patients get better with treatment, but some may experience neurological damage or permanent vision or hearing loss.

DID YOU KNOW? In 5 percent of female patients the condition occurs in connection with pregnancy or directly after giving birth.

EXTRA SOURCE: "Characteristics of Susac Syndrome: A Review of All Reported Cases," J. Dörr et al., *Nature Reviews Neurology*, 2013.

Systemic lupus erythematosus (SLE)

WHAT IS IT? The immune system attacks the connective tissue and other tissue, which results in inflammation. May affect the entire body, but most commonly affects the skin, joints, kidneys, blood, and nervous system. Incidence varies from country to country; in some areas the disease affects around one in every thousand inhabitants. Classic symptoms include a butterfly-shaped rash on the face, joint pain, and fever. Significant variation in symptoms, which fluctuate through periods in which they improve and worsen. With treatment many live a relatively normal life, but the condition may be extremely serious and life-threatening.

OTHER TYPES OF LUPUS: SLE is the most well known, but several other types of lupus also exist. Among these is drug-induced lupus, which goes away when the patient stops taking the relevant medication. Another variant is discoid lupus, which primarily affects the skin.

Systemic sclerosis (scleroderma)

WHAT IS IT? The immune system attacks the connective tissue, resulting in the formation of connective tissue in the skin, blood vessels, and internal organs. The skin becomes tighter, and organs may fail because the blood vessels become blocked. The prognosis varies, and the symptoms may remain mild and fairly stable over several years or rapidly worsen and take the patient's life. Treatment using stem cell transplantation has been attempted in serious cases. The results are promising, but there are serious risks associated with the procedure.

DID YOU KNOW? The word *scleroderma* stems from the Greek, and means "hard skin."

OTHER TYPES OF SCLERODERMA: CREST syndrome is a milder variant of systemic sclerosis, while localized scleroderma (morphea) is a variant that only affects the skin.

Temporal arteritis (giant cell arteritis)

WHAT IS IT? Inflammation of the blood vessels that affect the temporal artery and other blood vessels of the head and neck. The condition frequently occurs with polymyalgia rheumatica, and there is debate regarding whether these are actually two variants of the same disease. Almost never occurs in individuals below the age of fifty, and is most common in those over seventy. Visual disturbances, headache, and jaw pain are typical symptoms. Most patients become symptom-free through treatment with corticosteroids, but some may experience permanent vision loss.

DID YOU KNOW? Without treatment, the prognosis is poor. The disease may finally result in blindness, and in the worst case a fatal heart attack or stroke.

Tolosa-Hunt syndrome

WHAT IS IT? A condition that causes intense pain behind one of the eyes and may paralyze the eye muscles. The cause is unknown, but the area becomes inflamed, putting pressure on the nerves that control the muscles of the eye. Some researchers believe an autoimmune reaction to be the cause. The attack often passes by itself after a few weeks. With corticosteroids, the symptoms disappear over the course of two to three days. Around half of all patients experience recurrences.

DID YOU KNOW? The condition was first described in 1954. Just a few years later, doctors discovered the magical effect cortisone had on these patients, which is a sure sign that the diagnosis is correct.

Transverse myelitis

WHAT IS IT? Inflammation of the spinal cord. Often starts with sudden weakness in the muscles of the legs and occasionally the arms, urination problems, back pain, and sensory disturbances. May occur together with other autoimmune diseases but can also occur alone, often after an infection. The cause is unknown, but autoimmunity is suspected, and autoantibodies against proteins in the nervous system have been discovered. One-third of all patients recover, and another third experience mild aftereffects, while the final third develop serious aftereffects such as permanent weakness and spastic muscles.

EXTRA SOURCE: "Transverse Myelitis Fact Sheet," National Institute of Neurological Disorders and Stroke, ninds.nih.gov/Disorders/Patient-Caregiver-Education/Fact-Sheets/Transverse-Myelitis-Fact-Sheet.

Ulcerative colitis

WHAT IS IT? An inflammatory disease of the large intestine. Like Crohn's disease, it comes under the umbrella term of inflammatory bowel disease (IBD). In Western countries, around one in every thousand inhabitants has ulcerative colitis. Patients experience periods in which their symptoms improve and worsen. Stomach pain and bloody diarrhea are common, but for around half of all patients the symptoms are mild. In serious cases, the large intestines may be removed. Around one in every four patients experience symptoms outside the gut, such as inflamed joints, eye inflammation, rashes, and liver disease.

DID YOU KNOW? Patients with ulcerative colitis have an increased risk of bowel cancer.

Undifferentiated connective tissue disease (UCTD)

WHAT IS IT? Patients have symptoms of an autoimmune connective tissue disease but do not fulfil the criteria for one of the known variants, such as systemic lupus or scleroderma. The symptoms are often milder than in the other connective tissue diseases, although life-threatening complications may also occur in connection with UCTD.

DID YOU KNOW? For 20 to 40 percent of patients this is a temporary diagnosis. Those patients then receive a more specific diagnosis at a later date.

Vasculitis

WHAT IS IT? The immune system attacks the blood vessels, resulting in inflammation and circulatory failure in the affected area. May affect all kinds of blood vessels, and there are a number of subgroups of the disease, such as Kawasaki syndrome, Churg-Strauss syndrome, Wegener's disease, and Behcet's syndrome. Some types affect only children, while others only affect the elderly. The disease may be short-lived or lifelong. Most patients do well with treatment, but the condition can also be life-threatening.

DID YOU KNOW? The various types of vasculitis can affect both arteries and veins, and are defined by the size of the arteries affected. The main artery, the aorta, may also be attacked.

Vitiligo

WHAT IS IT? A skin disease in which white patches occur in the skin. The cells that produce the skin's pigment disappear, and researchers believe autoimmunity plays a role by attacking these cells. Affects 1–2 percent of the population. Often occurs in connection with other autoimmune diseases, such as type 1 diabetes and diseases of the thyroid gland. The condition is primarily a cosmetic problem, but for those who are severely affected this can be serious enough.

DID YOU KNOW? An extremely aggressive variant of vitiligo exists, in which 80 percent of the skin loses its pigmentation over the course of the year.

Vogt-Koyanagi-Harada disease

WHAT IS IT? An inflammatory disease that affects the pigmented parts of the eyes. May also affect the central nervous system, the middle ear, and the skin. More common in Asia and South America. The cause is unknown, but autoimmune reactions are thought to be involved. The disease has a variable progression, but may result in permanent vision loss. Early treatment with corticosteroids is important.

DID YOU KNOW? The disease's complex name is due to the fact that the disease was first regarded as different conditions, which were described by Vogt in 1906, Koyanagi in 1929, and Harada in 1926. These were later combined.

EXTRA SOURCE: "Vogt-Koyanagi-Haradas Sykdom," [Vogt-Koyanagi-Haradas disease] *Journal of the Norwegian Medical Association*, 2005.

WHAT DO WE KNOW ABOUT ENVIRONMENTAL FACTORS?

GENETIC PREDISPOSITION + triggering environmental factor = autoimmune disease. For example, a person with a genetic predisposition for celiac disease will first experience symptoms when eating gluten. A few environmental factors are proven to be a direct cause of specific diseases, but often the impact is broader, and an environmental factor increases the risk of several diseases. This is difficult to research, so in most cases we still know too little to say anything for sure.

GLUTEN. This is the classic example of an environmental factor we know is the cause of an autoimmune disease—celiac disease. The immune system reacts abnormally to gluten, and starts to attack the villi of the small intestine.

MEDICATIONS. Occasionally, medications may trigger autoimmune diseases. A known example is drug-induced lupus erythematosus (DILE), in which heart or blood pressure medications are often a triggering factor. The disease goes away when the patient stops taking the medicine.

SMOKING. The most certain risk factor for rheumatoid arthritis, particularly in patients with a certain type of genetic predisposition. Possibly also increases the risk of multiple sclerosis, systemic lupus, thyroiditis, Graves' disease, and Crohn's disease.

INFECTIONS. For several decades, viruses, bacteria, and parasites have been central suspected triggering factors in autoimmune diseases, but the connection is still largely unclear. The group A *Streptococcus* bacteria causes rheumatic fever and possibly also other autoimmune diseases. The virus that causes glandular fever, the Epstein-Barr virus (EBV), is also associated with several diseases.

CHEMICAL SUBSTANCES. Every day, we are exposed to many chemical substances through foods, makeup, detergents, plastic products, and so on. There are few studies on this, and much remains unclear. Silica, asbestos, and industrial solvents appear to increase the risk of certain autoimmune diseases. Some products used in hair dyes and nail cosmetics have also been studied, but without providing clear answers.

IONIZING RADIATION. Used in cancer treatments and X-rays. Radiotherapy appears to increase a patient's chances of developing autoimmune thyroiditis. A Swedish study showed that individuals exposed to such radiation at work were four times more likely to develop MS. Much remains unclear.

ULTRAVIOLET RADIATION (UV RAYS). Comes from the sun. The farther you live from the equator, the greater your risk of developing MS. Several studies show that exposure to sunlight protects against MS, and the amount of sunlight received before puberty may be crucial. Some studies have also found a connection between UV radiation and type 1 diabetes, rheumatoid arthritis, and vasculitis. Sunlight is an important source of vitamin D, and may be a factor in certain autoimmune diseases, particularly multiple sclerosis.

DIET. Autoimmune diseases are more common in rich, Western countries. Diet may be a risk factor. The results of studies differ, and much is unclear. One thing that has long been known is that fasting—not eating for a period of time—may help improve the condition of patients with rheumatoid arthritis.

OBESITY. Seems to increase the chances of developing diseases including rheumatoid arthritis, systemic lupus (SLE), psoriasis, and multiple sclerosis.

ENDOCRINE-DISRUPTING CHEMICALS. Chemical substances that affect the hormone system, especially estrogen. Found in items and substances such as plastic products, detergents, foods, and paints. A report by the World Health Organization (WHO) stated that it is reasonable to believe such substances may play a role in immunological diseases.

STRESS. A number of studies show that mental stress increases the chance of developing cardiovascular diseases and mental illnesses. The immune system is also affected, and chronic stress can lead to problems controlling inflammation. Stress may also worsen the progression of autoimmune diseases. One study showed an increased risk of autoimmune diseases among American soldiers suffering from post-traumatic stress disorder following terms of service in Afghanistan and Iraq.

TRAUMA. In the large American Adverse Childhood Experiences (ACE) Study, persons who had experienced childhood trauma had an increased risk of cardiovascular diseases, diseases of the liver, and depression—in addition to an increased risk of developing autoimmune diseases as adults. In another study, researchers found that individuals who had experienced childhood trauma had more inflammation in their bodies as adults.

Sources

IN 2010, A panel of experts reviewed the research on environmental factors and autoimmune diseases. The most important source of information is "Epidemiology of Environmental Exposures and Human Autoimmune Diseases: Findings From a National Institute of Environmental Health Sciences Expert Panel Workshop," F. W. Miller et al., *Journal of Autoimmunity*, 2012. Other sources are listed below.

"Sex-Specific Environmental Influences on the Development of Autoimmune Diseases," E. Tiniakou et al., *Clinical Immunology*, 2013.

"Human Autoimmune Diseases: A Comprehensive Update," L. Wang et al., *Journal of Internal Medicine*, 2015.

"The Role of Infections in Autoimmune Disease," A. M. Ercolini et al., *Clinical & Experimental Immunology*, 2009.

"Role of 'Western Diet' in Inflammatory Autoimmune Diseases," A. Manzel et al., *Current Allergy and Asthma Reports*, 2015.

"Obesity in Autoimmune Diseases: Not a Passive Bystander," M. Versini et al., *Autoimmunity Reviews*, 2014.

"State of the Science of Endocrine Disrupting Chemicals," Å. Bergman et al., WHO report, 2012.

"The Role of Environmental Estrogens and Autoimmunity," C. Chighizola et al., *Autoimmunity Reviews*, 2012.

"Cumulative Childhood Stress and Autoimmune Diseases in Adults," S. R. Dube et al., *Psychosomatic Medicine*, 2009.

"Childhood Maltreatment Predicts Adult Inflammation in a Life-Course Study," A. Danese et al., *Proceedings of the National Academies of Science*, 2007.

"Chronic Stress, Glucocorticoid Receptor Resistance, Inflammation, and Disease Risk," S. Cohen et al., *Proceedings of the National Academies of Science*, 2012.

"Psychological Stress and Disease," S. Cohen et al., JAMA, 2007.

"Elevated Risk for Autoimmune Disorders in Iraq and Afghanistan Veterans with Posttraumatic Stress Disorder," A. O'Donovan et al., *Biological Psychiatry*, 2015.

IMMUNE-SUPPRESSING
MEDICATIONS

GLUCOCORTICOIDS. Synthetically produced hormones that are similar to the hormone cortisol. May be administered in far greater doses than the body is able to produce itself. Often referred to as "cortisone" in everyday language. Available in a number of forms, including tablets, creams, inhalers, and injections.

METHOTREXATE. How this chemotherapy agent reduces the activity of autoimmune diseases is somewhat uncertain. Inhibits the T cells and reduces the production of a number of cytokines. In treating autoimmune diseases, a low dose is administered over a long period of time. Also often used in high doses in cancer treatments.

OTHER CHEMOTHERAPY AGENTS. Examples include cyclophosphamide, azathioprine, and mycophenolate. Used far less often than methotrexate.

ANTI-TNF (TNF INHIBITORS). Inhibit the cytokine TNF-alpha, a central signaling molecule in the inflammatory reaction. Often used in combination with methotrexate.

IL INHIBITORS. Interleukins (IL) are signaling molecules within the immune system. These medications inhibit various interleukins, such as IL-1, IL-6, IL-12, IL-17, and IL-23. Often prescribed for patients for whom anti-TNF and methotrexate have little effect.

ORENCIA. Affects the functioning of the T cells. Often prescribed for patients for whom anti-TNF and methotrexate have little effect.

B CELL DEPLETION THERAPY. Reduces the number of B cells—the cells that create antibodies—in the immune system. The most common drug is rituximab.

JAK INHIBITORS. Inhibit the Janus kinase (JAK) enzymes, thereby blocking the immune system's signaling pathways. A relatively new treatment that is used to treat rheumatoid arthritis, among other diseases.

SULFASALAZINE. Reduces inflammation and seems to inhibit bacteria. An old medication that is now less used than it once was.

LEFLUNOMIDE. Inhibits an enzyme, which results in the reduced production of certain immune cells (lymphocytes), and suppresses the immune reaction.

ANTIMALARIAL MEDICATIONS. Suppress the immune system. Are used in the treatment of some autoimmune diseases, such as systemic lupus (SLE) and rheumatoid arthritis.

CYCLOSPORINE. Inhibits the production of IL-2 and the growth of T cells. Also used to prevent the rejection of transplanted organs.

GOLD. Once frequently used in the treatment of rheumatoid arthritis and still in use today, although far more rarely. The mechanism by which it works is still unknown.

Other treatments that affect the immune system

INTRAVENOUS IMMUNOGLOBULIN THERAPY (IVIG). Immuno-globins are antibodies. Patients are administered antibodies from the blood of healthy donors, which helps in the treatment of some autoimmune diseases.

PLASMAPHERESIS. A method of cleaning the blood, performed in hospital. The blood cells are separated from the plasma (fluid), and the plasma is replaced. This makes it possible to remove harmful antibodies from the blood.

STEM CELL TRANSPLANTATION. There are two types: The first alternative involves destroying the body's stem cells in the bone marrow and then transplanting new ones from a donor. The second option is to extract stem cells from the patient, then return them to the patient's body following the removal of malfunctioning immune cells (autologous stem cell transplantation).

SOURCES

About the patients in the book: In the stories about Marit and Jan I have used their real first names in accordance with their wishes. In the stories about Linda, Peter, Eva, and Sandra, I haven't used the patients' real names.

Prologue

. . . over a hundred diseases are thought to be caused by the body's own soldiers making disastrous mistakes: This is a question of definition, since there are no clear limits as to what may be classified as an autoimmune disease. Researchers often used to say that there are over eighty autoimmune diseases, but in recent years more have been added to the list, and many now believe there to be well over one hundred. The American Autoimmune Related Diseases Association lists over 140 diseases: aarda.org/diseaselist/.

In an article from 2012, researchers characterize eighty-one diseases as autoimmune: "Updated Assessment of the Prevalence, Spectrum and Case Definition of Autoimmune Disease," S. M. Hayter et al., *Autoimmunity Reviews*, August 2012.

Chapter 1: Beginnings

. . . the immunological paradox of pregnancy: "The Immunology of Successful Pregnancy," A. L. Veenstra van Nieuwenhoven et al., *Human Reproduction Update*, 2003.

...bleak economic times: Information about the economic situation in Liverpool in the 1980s is taken from the English Wikipedia article about the city.

Chapter 2: The Master and a Clue

Around one in every hundred people will develop rheumatoid arthritis: According to Medscape and BMJ Best Practice, around 1 percent of the population is affected by rheumatoid arthritis, but incidence varies by country and ethnicity.

When the Dutch artist Rubens painted *The Three Graces* in 1635: "Historical Perspectives on the Etiology of Rheumatoid Arthritis," B. S. Pouya Entzami et al., *Hand Clinics*, February 2011.

Charaka... wrote about patients who experienced pain, stiffness, and shrinkage in the joints: "Evidence of Rheumatoid Arthritis in Ancient India," R. D. Sturrock et al., *Arthritis and Rheumatism*, January 1977.

...credit the French surgeon Augustin Jacob Landré-Beauvais (entire section):
1. Pouya Entzami et al., "Historical Perspectives on the Etiology of Rheumatoid Arthritis."
2. *Intolerant Bodies: A Short History of Autoimmunity*, Warwick Anderson and Ian R. Mackay, Johns Hopkins University Press, 2014.

Every tenth patient suffers such a severe case of the disease that they may become markedly disabled: Norwegian Health Informatics (database), nhi.no/sykdommer/muskel-skjelett/giktsykdommer/leddgikt-oversikt/?page=6.

...among the leading causes of death in the world, particularly for young and middle-aged women:
1. "Autoimmune Diseases: A Leading Cause of Death Among Young and Middle-Aged Women in the United States," S. J. Walsh et al., *American Journal of Public Health*, September 2000.
2. "Burden of Mortality Associated With Autoimmune Diseases Among Females in the United Kingdom," S. L. Thomas et al., *American Journal of Public Health*, November 2010.

... **survey of eighty-three women with rheumatoid arthritis:** "Hypothalamic-Pituitary-Gonadal Axis Variations Associated With the Onset of Rheumatoid Arthritis," A. S. Kåss et al., EULAR abstract, Barcelona, 2007.

... **reading the available reports, and my suspicions were soon confirmed:** Sources from my doctorate, "Gonadotropin-Releasing Hormone Antagonism: A Potential Pathway for Anti-Inflammatory Treatment in Rheumatoid Arthritis," A. Kåss, Faculty of Medicine, University of Oslo, 2014. Some examples:

1. "Maternal-Fetal Disparity in HLA Class II Alloantigens and the Pregnancy-Induced Amelioration of Rheumatoid Arthritis," J. L. Nelson et al., *New England Journal of Medicine*, August 1993.

2. "Effect of Pregnancy and Hormonal Changes on the Activity of Rheumatoid Arthritis," M. Østensen et al., *Scandinavian Journal of Rheumatology*, 1983.

3. "The Role of Pregnancy in the Course and Aetiology of Rheumatoid Arthritis," J. A. Da Silva, *Clinical Rheumatology*, 1992.

4. "Onset of Symptoms of Rheumatoid Arthritis in Relation to Age, Sex and Menopausal Transition," S. Goemaere et al., *Journal of Rheumatology*, 1990.

Chapter 3: Nature Versus Nurture

... **a line estimated to be twice the diameter of our solar system:** There are several sources for this calculation, including "How Long Is Your DNA?," Hannah Ashworth, *Science Focus* (BBC), sciencefocus.com/qa/how-long-your-dna.

In the year 2000, researchers from the international Human Genome Project presented the result: Press release from the White House in June 2000. A rough draft of the human genome was presented before researchers presented a complete version in 2003. web.ornl.gov/sci/techresources/Human_Genome/project/clinton1.shtml.

... **around twenty thousand functional genes:** Functional genes are genes that code for proteins—how many there are continues to be disputed. Sources include the following articles:

1. "Human Genome Is Much More Than Just Genes," E. Pennisi, *Science Magazine*, September 2012.

2. "The Dark Side of the Human Genome," K. R. Chi, *Nature*, August 17, 2016.

3. "Eukaryotic Genome Complexity," L. Pray, *Nature Education*, 2008.

. . . around the same number as in a millimeter-long roundworm:

1. "A Journey Into the Genome: What's There?" H. Gee, *Nature*, February 2001.

2. Wikipedia article about the roundworm *C. elegans*.

3. Great Norwegian Encyclopedia (online) article about genes.

. . . on average, there is around a 30 percent chance that the second twin will develop the same disease: From a report by the National Institutes of Health (NIH) in 2005: "Progress in Autoimmune Disease Research."

. . . my risk of developing the disease is around three times greater than that of others: "Familial Risks and Heritability of Rheumatoid Arthritis: Role of Rheumatoid Factor/Anti-Citrullinated Protein Antibody Status, Number and Type of Affected Relatives, Sex, and Age," T. Frisell et al., *Arthritis & Rheumatology*, November 2013.

. . . where you live is a decisive factor in your risk of becoming ill: Incidence figures throughout this section are taken from "The Global Burden of Rheumatoid Arthritis: Estimates From the Global Burden of Disease 2010 Study," M. Cross et al., *Annals of the Rheumatic Diseases*, February 2014.

. . . had a risk of developing MS that was three times greater than that of their parents who had moved to Norway as adults: "Prevalence of Multiple Sclerosis Among Immigrants in Norway," P. Berg-Hansen et al., *Multiple Sclerosis*, May 2015.

. . . the same trend can be seen for a number of other autoimmune diseases:

1. "Environmental Risk Factors for Type 1 Diabetes," M. Rewers et al., *Lancet*, June 2016.

2. "Environmental Risk Factors for Inflammatory Bowel Diseases: Evidence Based Literature Review," A. T. Abegunde et al., *World Journal of Gastroenterology*, July 2016.

. . . my chances of developing rheumatoid arthritis increased: This study is from Sweden and shows that children of certain immigrants have a higher risk of developing rheumatoid arthritis than their parents who moved to Sweden as adults. "Risks of Rheumatic Diseases in First- and Second-Generation Immigrants in Sweden: A Nationwide Follow Up Study," X. Li et al., *Arthritis & Rheumatology*, June 2009.

Our genes are responsible for around half the risk of developing rheumatoid arthritis, while environmental factors stand for the rest: "Characterizing the Quantitative Genetic Contribution to Rheumatoid Arthritis Using Data From Twins," A. J. MacGregor et al., *Arthritis and Rheumatism*, January 2000.

. . . far greater chance of developing rheumatoid arthritis if you smoke—but only if you also have a genetic predisposition for the disease:

1. "Impact of Smoking as a Risk Factor for Developing Rheumatoid Arthritis: A Meta-Analysis of Observational Studies," D. Sugiyama et al., *Annals of the Rheumatic Diseases*, 2010.

2. "Gene-Environment Interaction Between the DRB1 Shared Epitope and Smoking in the Risk of Anti-Citrullinated Protein Antibody-Positive Rheumatoid Arthritis: All Alleles Are Important," E. Lundström et al., *Arthritis and Rheumatism*, 2009.

Chapter 4: A Dance out of the Wheelchair

The story of Philip Hench is taken from the following sources:

1. His Nobel Prize lecture from 1950: "The Reversibility of Certain Rheumatic and Non-Rheumatic Conditions by the Use of Cortisone or of the Pituitary Adrenocorticotropic Hormone."

2. Obituary for Philip Hench in *Rheumatology* 5, 2002, by M. Lloyd.

3. "Cortisone, 1949: A Year in the Political Life of a Drug," H. M. Marks, *Bulletin of the History of Medicine*, 1992.

4. "The Discovery of Cortisone: A Personal Memory," J. H. Glyn, *British Medical Journal*, September 1998.

5. "The Discovery and Early Use of Cortisone," J. Glyn, *Journal of The Royal Society of Medicine*, December 1997.

6. "Diamonds Are Forever: The Cortisone Legacy," S. G. Hillier, *Journal of Endocrinology*, 2007.

7. *The Rise and Fall of Modern Medicine*, James Le Fanu, Abacus, 2011.

"It would be gratifying if one were able to repeat nature's miracle," wrote Hench: The quotation is taken from sources 2 and 7 in the list above.

During the Second World War, rumors were circulating about German pilots: The information about German pilots and Argentinian cattle is taken from sources 2, 5, 6, and 7 in the list above.

Hench was given five grams: Source 2 in the list above.

His selected test patient was Mrs. Gardner: Sources 2 and 7 in the list above.

When Hench presented his results for the first time, in April 1949: Sources 2 and 3 in the list above.

He'd ended up in the hormone system (about the HPA-immune axis and the immune system): "The HPA-Immune Axis and the Immunomodulatory Actions of Glucocorticoids in the Brain," M. A. Bellavance et al., *Frontiers in Immunology*, March 2014.

As the birth draws near, pregnant women have two to three times more cortisol in their bodies than usual: "A Longitudinal Study of Plasma and Urinary Cortisol in Pregnancy and Postpartum," C. Jung et al., *Journal of Clinical Endocrinology & Metabolism*, May 2011.

...estrogen that captured my interest: Sources from my doctorate, Kåss, "Gonadotropin-Releasing Hormone Antagonism." Some examples:

1. "Estrogens and Arthritis," M. Cutolo et al., *Rheumatic Diseases Clinics of North America*, February 2005.

2. "Endocrine End-Points in Rheumatoid Arthritis," L. Castagnetta et al., *Annals of the New York Academy of Sciences*, June 1999.

3. "Role of Oestrogen in the Development of Joint Symptoms?" A. L. Tan et al., *Lancet Oncology*, September 2008.

. . . Turner syndrome:

1. Some facts taken from Norwegian Health Informatics (database): nhi.no/sykdommer/barn/arvelige-og-medfodte-tilstander/turners-syndrom/.
2. "Autoimmune Diseases in Women With Turner's Syndrome," K. T. Jørgensen et al., *Arthritis and Rheumatism*, March 2010.

Chapter 5: The Lonely Researcher

In the United States, over twenty million people live with such illnesses—for comparison, around fifteen million people live with a cancer diagnosis:

1. Report from the National Institutes of Health (NIH) in 2005: "Progress in Autoimmune Disease Research."
2. The number of patients living with a cancer diagnosis: cancer.gov/about-cancer/understanding/statistics.

Still, health authorities have allocated ten times as much funding to cancer research as to research into autoimmune diseases: Statistics from the American Autoimmune Related Diseases Association, aarda.org/news-information/statistics/. Figures are from 2003: US$591 million per year for autoimmune diseases versus US$6.1 billion for cancer.

Chapter 6: The Body at War

Primary sources for this chapter include:

1. *How the Immune System Works*, Lauren M. Sompayrac, Wiley-Blackwell, 2015.
2. *Immunity*, William E. Paul, Johns Hopkins University Press, 2015.
3. Articles about the immune system and associated cell types from *Encyclopaedia Britannica*.
4. Background material from several studies and articles about the immune system.

Every second, the bone marrow creates more than two million red blood cells: Source 1 in the list above.

If we were to lay it out flat, the skin would cover about 20 square feet . . . but the internal surfaces of the mucous membranes would cover an area of almost 4,300 square feet: Source 1 in the list above.

The body produces around one hundred billion of these foot soldiers every day (neutrophil granulocytes): "Neutrophil," *Encyclopaedia Britannica.*

They can even make their own cobweblike substances: "Neutrophil Extracellular Traps in Immunity and Disease," V. Papayannopoulos, *Nature Reviews Immunology*, February 2018.

Similar mechanisms probably existed in the first multicellular organisms to arise: "On the Origin of the Immune System," J. Travis, *Science*, May 2009.

It's like the old rice and chessboard story: The legend exists in many versions as an example of exponential growth. The comparison to Mount Everest is highlighted in several sources, including in the book *The Second Machine Age* by Erik Brynjolfsson and Andrew McAfee, psmag.com/economics/the-economic-geography-of-the-second-machine-age.

. . . around three hundred billion T cells and three billion B cells: Sompayrac, *How the Immune System Works.*

. . . soon an army of clones is mobilized: Paul, *Immunity.*

The rare IPEX syndrome: "Immunodysregulation Polyendocrinopathy Enteropathy X-Linked Syndrome (IPEX)," T. Banks, Medscape, 2016.

B cells . . . B for the bone marrow: The "B" originally comes from the organ "bursa of Fabricius" in birds, where the B cells were first discovered and called "bursa-derived cells." When the B cells were found in the bone marrow in humans, they were named "bone-marrow-derived cells." See "The Early History of B Cells," M. D. Cooper, *Nature Reviews Immunology*, 2015.

TNF... holds a senior position among the cytokines and manages important parts of the inflammatory response:

1. "TNF-Mediated Inflammatory Disease," J. R. Bradley, *Journal of Pathology*, December 2007.
2. "Pathogenetic Insights From the Treatment of Rheumatoid Arthritis," I. B. McInnes et al., *Lancet*, June 2017.

Chapter 7: An Autoimmune Attack

Research from the United States and United Kingdom shows that autoimmune diseases are among the top ten causes of death for women under the age of sixty-five:

1. Walsh et al., "Autoimmune Diseases: A Leading Cause of Death Among Young and Middle-Aged Women in the United States."
2. Thomas et al., "Burden of Mortality Associated With Autoimmune Diseases Among Females in the United Kingdom."

Sources for the history of autoimmunity:

1. *A History of Immunology*, Arthur M. Silverstein, Academic Press, 1989.
2. Anderson and Mackay, *Intolerant Bodies*.
3. "The Rise and Fall of Horror Autotoxicus and Forbidden Clones," J. Charles Jennette et al., *Kidney International*, September 2010.

Over a hundred years ago the medical literature was full of: Anderson and Mackay, *Intolerant Bodies*.

A study published in the journal *Lancet* in 2009: "Incidence Trends for Childhood Type 1 Diabetes in Europe During 1989–2003 and Predicted New Cases 2005–20: A Multicentre Prospective Registration Study," C. C. Patterson et al., *Lancet*, June 2009.

In 2005, twice as many Finnish children developed the disease: "Time Trends in the Incidence of Type 1 Diabetes in Finnish Children: A Cohort Study," V. Harjutsalo et al., *Lancet*, May 2008.

Fewer people seem to be developing rheumatoid arthritis than previously: "The Changing Face of Rheumatoid Arthritis: Why the Decline in Incidence," A. J. Silman, *Arthritis & Rheumatism*, March 2002. Whether there has been an actual decrease in the number of cases of rheumatoid arthritis is contentious, since some studies have also shown that the incidence is the same as in previous years. See, for example: Cross et al., "The Global Burden of Rheumatoid Arthritis: Estimates From the Global Burden of Disease 2010 Study."

. . . despite the decrease in some autoimmune diseases, the overall trend is that an increasing number of individuals are developing them: Report from the National Institutes of Health (NIH) in 2005: *Progress in Autoimmune Disease Research.*

Information about rheumatic fever is from Norwegian Health Informatics (database) and Wikipedia: nhi.no/sykdommer/hjertekar/ulike-sykdommer/ gikt-feber/; en.wikipedia.org/wiki/Rheumatic_fever.

. . . across the world, over 300,000 people die from rheumatic fever: "Global, Regional and National Burden of Rheumatic Heart Disease, 1990–2015," D. A. Watkins et al., *New England Journal of Medicine*, August 2017.

In the late 1970s, a group of researchers discovered: "Fetal Cells in the Blood of Pregnant Women. Detection and Enrichment by Fluorescence-Activated Cell Sorting," L. A. Herzenberg et al., *Proceedings of the National Academy of Sciences*, March 1979.

Some of the fetal cells continue to live in the mother for years afterward:
1. "Pregnancy and the Risk of Autoimmune Disease," A. S. Khashan et al., *PLoS One*, 2011.
2. "Beyond Birth: A Child's Cells May Help or Harm the Mother Long After Delivery," N. Chute, *Scientific American*, April 30, 2010.
3. "A Pregnancy Souvenir: Cells That Are Not Your Own," Carl Zimmer, *New York Times*, September 10, 2015.
4. "Gender Differences in Autoimmune Disease," S. T. Ngo et al., *Frontiers in Neuroendocrinology*, May 2014.

"The good bacteria" section is based on the following sources:

1. "Microbiome: Puppy Power," S. Gupta, *Nature*, March 29, 2017.
2. "Cleaning Up the Hygiene Hypothesis," M. Scudellari, *Proceedings of the National Academy of Sciences*, February 14, 2017.
3. "Questions Persist: Environmental Factors in Autoimmune Disease," C. W. Schmidt, *Environmental Health Perspectives*, June 2011.
4. "Allergies: An Inflammatory Subject," Festschrift of the British Society for Immunology, October 2016.
5. "Unraveling the Hygiene Hypothesis of Helminthes and Autoimmunity: Origins, Pathophysiology, and Clinical Applications," M. Versini et al., BMC *Medicine*, 2015.
6. "Human Microbiome," *Encyclopaedia Britannica*.
7. "Role of the Microbiota in Immunity and Inflammation," Y. Belkaid et al., *Cell*, March 2014.
8. "Microbiota: Hidden Communities of Friends and Foes," Festschrift of the British Society for Immunology, October 2016.
9. "Does the Microbiota Play a Role in the Pathogenesis in Autoimmune Diseases?" M. H. McLean et al., *Gut*, November 2014.

...in 1989, when the hygiene hypothesis was put forth: "Hay Fever, Hygiene and Household Size," D. P. Strachan, *British Medical Journal*, November 1989.

...we have several thousand billion cells in our bodies, but the number of bacteria we contain is at least equally vast: There are a number of estimates regarding the number of cells and microorganisms in the body, and all of them are uncertain. In a study from 2016, researchers estimated that a man with a height of 170 centimeters weighing 70 kilos (about 5'7" and 155 pounds) has around thirty billion cells in his body and thirty-nine billion bacteria (a billion is one thousand million). However, the researchers also emphasized that there are significant variations from person to person. See "Scientists Bust Myth That Our Bodies Have More Bacteria Than Human Cells," A. Abbott, *Science*, January 2016.

...**theory known as the "old friends" hypothesis:** "Mycobacteria and Other Environmental Organisms as Immunomodulators for Immunoregulatory Disorders," G. A. Rook et al., *Springer Seminars in Immunopathology*, February 2004.

Studies show that people in more developed countries have less varied bacterial flora than people in poorer countries:

1. "Distinct Distal Gut Microbiome Diversity and Composition in Healthy Children From Bangladesh and the United States," A. Lin et al., *PLoS One*, January 2013.
2. "Human Gut Microbiome Viewed Across Age and Geography," T. Yatsunenko et al., *Nature*, May 2012.

Both human and animal studies indicate that different bacterial flora both increase and reduce the risk of autoimmune diseases:

1. "The Gut Microbiota in Immune-Mediated Inflammatory Diseases," J. D. Forbes, *Frontiers in Microbiology*, July 2016.
2. "Multiple Sclerosis: What's It Got to Do With Your Gut?" A. Burton, *Lancet Neurology*, December 2017.

In recent years, studies have shown that a quarter of patients with ulcerative colitis:

1. "Fecal Microbiota Transplantation Induces Remission in Patients With Active Ulcerative Colitis in a Randomized Controlled Trial," P. Moayyedi et al., *Gastroenterology*, July 2015.
2. "Multidonor Intensive Faecal Microbiota Transplantation for Active Ulcerative Colitis: A Randomised Placebo-Controlled Trial," S. Paramsothy et al., *Lancet*, March 2017.

Researchers have also tested it on female mice made susceptible to type 1 diabetes: "Sex Differences in the Gut Microbiome Drive Hormone-Dependent Regulation of Autoimmunity," J. G. M. Markle et al., *Science*, March 2013.

The "Terror in the joints" section is largely based on my own doctoral thesis and the sources listed therein: Kåss, "Gonadotropin-Releasing Hormone

Antagonism." The following is also a central source of information regarding the disease mechanism in rheumatoid arthritis: "The Pathogenesis of Rheumatoid Arthritis," I. B. McInnes et al., *New England Journal of Medicine*, December 2011.

The glandular fever virus is called the Epstein-Barr virus: "Epstein-Barr Virus in Systemic Autoimmune Diseases," A. H. Draborg et al., *Clinical and Developmental Immunology*, 2013.

But there is one strain of bacteria that seems to be connected to rheumatoid arthritis:

1. "Mouth and Other Bacteria May Trigger RA," Arthritis Foundation.
2. "Periodontal Disease and Rheumatoid Arthritis: The Evidence Accumulates for Complex Pathobiologic Interactions," C. O. Bingham et al., *Current Opinion in Rheumatology*, May 2013.
3. "Aggregatibacter Actinomycetemcomitans-Induced Hypercitrullination Links Periodontal Infection to Autoimmunity in Rheumatoid Arthritis," M. F. Konig et al., *Science Translational Medicine*, 2016.

Perhaps the most famous example of this was in 1928, when Alexander Fleming: "Alexander Fleming," Wikipedia, en.wikipedia.org/wiki/Alexander_Fleming.

Another example is the American farmer who in 1933: *Karl Paul Link. A Biographical Memoir*, Robert H. Burris, National Academy of Sciences, 1994.

Chapter 8: Judgment Day

My study was small, and the first of its kind: See "The Association of Luteinizing Hormone and Follicle-Stimulating Hormone With Cytokines and Markers of Disease Activity in Rheumatoid Arthritis: A Case-Control Study," A. S. Kåss et al., *Scandinavian Journal of Rheumatology*, March 2010.

The example of estrogen supplements and heart disease is from the following sources:

1. "The Hormone Replacement–Coronary Heart Disease Conundrum: Is This the Death of Observational Epidemiology?" D. A. Lawlor et al., *International Journal of Epidemiology*, June 2004.

2. "Hormone Replacement Therapy and Your Heart," Mayo Clinic, 2015.

3. "Menopausal Hormone Therapy and Heart Disease," National Heart, Lung and Blood Institute, 2012.

4. "Lessons Learned From the Women's Health Initiative Trials of Menopausal Hormone Therapy," J. E. Rossouw et al., *Obstetrics and Gynecology*, January 2013.

5. *Epidemiology Kept Simple: An Introduction to Traditional and Modern Epidemiology*, B. Burt Gerstman, Wiley-Blackwell, 2013.

6. "Postmenopausal Hormone Replacement Therapy and the Primary Prevention of Cardiovascular Disease," L. L. Humphrey et al., *Annals of Internal Medicine*, August 2002.

The effects of hormone replacement on heart disease continue to be much discussed, and some studies indicate that when women start taking such medications is a critical factor affecting the risk of heart diseases. Younger women seem to experience positive effects of hormone replacement therapy when menopause sets in. See "Where Are We 10 Years After the Women's Health Initiative?" T. A. Lobo, *Journal of Clinical Endocrinology and Metabolism*, May 2013.

Chapter 9: The Female Diseases

Many of the sources used in the writing of this chapter come from my doctoral thesis. Some are specified below, but additional studies can be found in the references section of my thesis: Kåss, "Gonadotropin-Releasing Hormone Antagonism." The following article is another important source for this chapter: "Effects of Menopause on Autoimmune Diseases," M. A. Farage et al., *Expert Reviews of Obstetrics & Gynecology*, 2012.

SOURCES

"Sex differences in autoimmune diseases have long been known": E. I. Tiniakou et al., "Sex-Specific Environmental Influences on the Development of Autoimmune Diseases," *Clinical Immunology*, November 2013.

Of every hundred patients suffering from an autoimmune disease, around eighty of them will be women: "Sex Differences in Autoimmune Disease From a Pathological Perspective," L. D. Fairweather et al., *American Journal of Pathology*, September 2008.

A Swedish study shows that women have a greater risk of developing rheumatoid arthritis if they enter menopause before the age of forty-five.: "Early Menopause Is an Independent Predictor of Rheumatoid Arthritis," M. Pikwer et al., *Annals of Rheumatic Diseases*, March 2012.

Women suffering from lupus find that their condition worsens during pregnancy: Farage, "Effects of Menopause on Autoimmune Diseases."

. . . administering estrogen to patients suffering from rheumatoid arthritis might ease the symptoms: "Effect of Oestrogen Treatment on Clinical and Laboratory Manifestations of Rheumatoid Arthritis," J. W. Bijlsma et al., *Annals of the Rheumatic Diseases*, 1987.

. . . little or no improvement from increased estrogen: "Effects of Postmenopausal Hormone Therapy on Rheumatoid Arthritis: The Women's Health Initiative Randomized Controlled Trials," B. Walitt et al., *Arthritis and Rheumatism*, 2008.

. . . hoped that the contraceptive pill might protect women against rheumatoid arthritis:
1. "Reduction in Incidence of Rheumatoid Arthritis Associated With Oral Contraceptives," S. J. Wingrave et al., *Lancet*, 1978.
2. "Diminished Incidence of Severe Rheumatoid Arthritis Associated With Oral Contraceptive Use," D. van Zeben et al., *Arthritis and Rheumatism*, 1990.

About the hypothalamus, pituitary gland, and GnRH:

1. Sources from my doctoral thesis: Kåss, "Gonadotropin-Releasing Hormone Antagonism."

2. "Hypothalamus," Great Norwegian Encyclopedia (online).

3. "Hypothalamus," *Encyclopaedia Britannica*.

... **Prader-Willi syndrome:** From Norwegian Health Informatics (database): nhi.no/sykdommer/barn/arvelige-og-medfodte-tilstander/prader-willi-syndrom/.

Every year, *Forbes* magazine lists the world's largest companies: "Global 2000: The World's Largest Public Companies," *Forbes*. Pfizer, Novartis, Roche, Sanofi, and Merck are all among the world's one hundred biggest companies on the *Forbes* list for 2017. Johnson & Johnson is the biggest of all, but is not just a pharmaceutical company.

Chapter 10: Gold, Mustard Gas, and the World's Most Valuable Medicine

... **a sixty-two-year-old British woman became the basis for an experiment:** "Do Gold Rings Protect Against Articular Erosion in Rheumatoid Arthritis?" D. M. Mulherin et al., *Annals of the Rheumatic Diseases*, August 1997.

About the use of gold and sulfasalazine:

1. "Rheumatoid Arthritis Treatments: A Historical Perspective," D. Aggarwal et al., *JSM Arthritis*, July 2016.

2. "Medical Uses of Gold Compounds: Past, Present and Future," S. P. Pricker, *Gold Bulletin*, 1996.

Sources about the discovery of methotrexate:

1. "Methotrexate in Rheumatoid Arthritis: A Quarter Century of Development," M. E. Weinblatt, *Transactions of the American Clinical and Climatological Association*, 2013.

2. "The Birth of Cancer Therapy: Accident and Research," N. Godoy, Pan American Health Organization/WHO.

3. "Mustard Agents," Organisation for the Prohibition of Chemical Weapons.

4. *The Emperor of All Maladies: A Biography of Cancer*, Siddhartha Mukherjee, Simon & Schuster, 2010.
5. Anderson and Mackay, *Intolerant Bodies*.

Sources about the discovery of anti-TNF:
1. "Bench to Bedside: Research and Development of Anti-TNF Therapy" (video), Ravinder Maini, January 31, 2011, youtube.com/watch?v=ZAEiP_9Ltkc.
2. "Treatment of Rheumatoid Arthritis With Chimeric Monoclonal Antibodies to Tumour Necrosis Factor Alpha," M. J. Elliot et al., *Arthritis and Rheumatism*, December 1993.
3. "Randomised Double-Blind Comparison of Chimeric Monoclonal Antibody to Tumour Necrosis Factor Alpha (CA2) Versus Placebo in Rheumatoid Arthritis," M. J. Elliot et al., *Lancet*, October 1994.
4. *Love and Science: A Memoir*, Jan Vilcek, Seven Stories Press, 2016.

On the list of the world's top-selling pharmaceuticals for 2016: "The Top 15 Best-Selling Drugs of 2016," *Genetic Engineering & Bio-technology News*, March 6, 2017.

. . . on a par with the yearly revenue of Nike: "The World's Biggest Public Companies," *Forbes* Global 2000, 2017.

Chapter 11: Going Against the Stream

The story about Barry Marshall is based on his biography on the Nobel Prize website: nobelprize.org/nobel_prizes/medicine/laureates/2005/marshall-bio.html.

Chapter 12: A Nobel Prize Winner Answers the Phone

The story of the discovery of GnRH is mainly based on the following sources:
1. *The Nobel Duel*, Nicholas Wade, Anchor Press/Doubleday, 1981.
2. Biographies and Nobel Lectures of the researchers on nobelprize.org.
3. "Hypothalamic Control of Anterior Pituitary Function: A History," H. Charlton, *Journal of Neuroendocrinology*, 2008.

About GnRH:

1. Sources from my doctoral thesis: Kåss, "Gonadotropin-Releasing Hormone Antagonism."
2. "Gonadotropin-Releasing Hormone," *Encyclopedia Britannica.*
3. "Molecular Biology of Gonadotropin-Releasing Hormone (GnRH)-I, GnRH-II, and Their Receptors in Humans," C. K. Cheng et al., *Endocrine Reviews*, April 2005.

About lampreys:

1. "Meet a Lamprey. Your Ancestors," BBC, November 2015.
2. "A Lamprey From the Devonian Period of South Africa," R. W. Gess et al., *Nature*, October 2006.
3. "The Interrelationship of Estrogen Receptor and GnRH in a Basal Vertebrate, the Sea Lamprey," S. A. Sower et al., *Frontiers in Endocrinology*, October 2011.
4. "The Origins of the Vertebrate Hypothalamic-Pituitary-Gonadal (HPG) and Hypothalamic-Pituitary-Thyroid (HPT) Endocrine Systems: New Insights From Lampreys," S. A. Sower et al., *General and Comparative Endocrinology*, March 2009.

In 1980, Richard M. Sharpe pointed out this phenomenon in an article published in *Nature*: "Extra-Pituitary Actions of LHRH and its Agonists," R. M. Sharpe, *Nature*, July 1980.

... studies show that patients with multiple sclerosis have an increased risk of relapse:

1. "Increase in Multiple Sclerosis Activity After Assisted Reproduction Technology," J. Correale et al., *Annals of Neurology*, 2012.
2. "Increased MS Relapse Rate During Assisted Reproduction Technique," K. Hellwig et al., *Journal of Neurology*, 2008.
3. "Increase in Multiple Sclerosis Relapse Rate Following In Vitro Fertilization," D. A. Lapalud et al., *Neurology*, 2006.

In a study undertaken on mice with induced lupus: "Modulation of the Expression of Murine Lupus by Gonadotropin-Releasing Hormone Analogs," J. D. Jacobson et al., *Endocrinology*, June 1994.

. . . seemed to protect the mice from developing type 1 diabetes: "Modulation of Diabetes With Gonadotropin-Releasing Hormone Antagonists in the Nonobese Mouse Model of Autoimmune Diabetes," A. Mansoor et al., *Endocrinology*, January 2004.

In patients with prostate cancer, it has been observed that those who are given GnRH inhibitors are less likely to develop cardiovascular disease: "Lower Risk of Cardiovascular Events and Death in Men Receiving ADT by Gonadotropin Releasing Hormone Antagonist, Degarelix, Compared With Luteinising Hormone-Releasing Agonists," B. Tombal et al., article presented at The European Association of Urology 28th Annual Congress, Milan, Italy, 2013.

Chapter 14: The Experiment

According to an American survey: The survey was undertaken by the American Autoimmune Related Diseases Association. Over 45 percent of those asked experienced being perceived as "chronic complainers" before they were diagnosed: aarda.org/who-we-help/patients/women-and-autoimmunity/.

The information about ankylosing spondylitis and HLA-B27 was obtained from Health Norway (helsenorge.no): helsenorge.no/sykdom/muskel-og-skjelett/bekhterevs-sykdom.

About lupus and antimalarial medications:
1. "The Role of Antimalarial Agents in the Treatment of SLE and Lupus Nephritis," S. J. Lee et al., *Nature Reviews Nephrology*, December 2011.
2. "Plaquenil: From Malaria Treatment to Managing Lupus," *The Rheumatologist*, May 15, 2015.
3. "The History of Lupus," Lupus Foundation of America.

. . . only around four in ten patients experienced any improvement: "Golimumab in Patients With Active Rheumatoid Arthritis After Treatment

With Tumour Necrosis Factor Alpha Inhibitors (GO-AFTER study): A Multi-centre, Randomised, Double-Blind, Placebo-Controlled, Phase III Trial," J. S. Smolen et al., *Lancet*, July 2009.

Chapter 15: The Billion-Dollar Companies Arrive

About Ferring Pharmaceuticals: "Our History," on Ferring's website: ferring.com/en/about-ferring/our-history/.

Epilogue: The Search for a Longer Life

The epilogue is based on the following sources:

1. "Evolution of the Immune System in Humans From Infancy to Old Age," A. K. Simon et al., *Proceedings: Biological Sciences*, 2015.
2. "Immunosenescence: Emerging Challenges for an Ageing Population," D. Aw et al., *Immunology*, April 2007.

Researchers have stimulated GnRH production in rats and observed that the thymus grows:

1. "Effect of GnRH Agonists on the Thymus in Female Rats," K. M. Ataya et al., *Acta Endocrinologia*, December 1989.
2. A. Mansoor et al., "Modulation of Diabetes With Gonadotropin-Releasing Hormone Antagonists in the Nonobese Mouse Model of Autoimmune Diabetes."

INDEX